I0096446

Chronic Pain
Journal for
Calm

Arielle Haughee

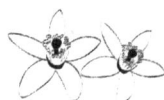

ORANGE BLOSSOM
PUBLISHING

Maitland, Florida

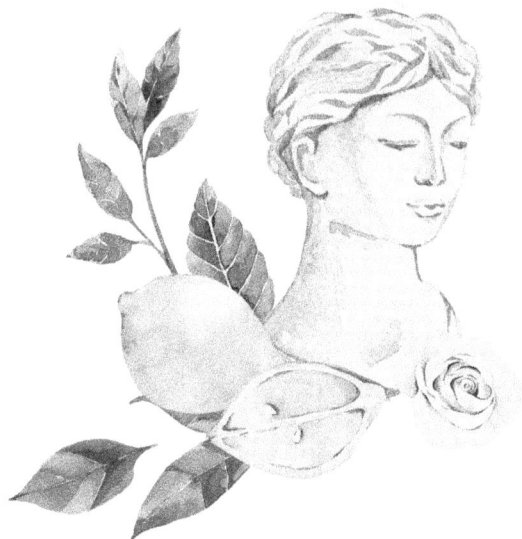

© 2022 by Arielle Haughee.
All rights reserved. No part of this book may be transmitted in any form or by any means, electronic or mechanical, including photocopying, recording, or by any information storage or retrieval system, in part, in any form, without the permission of the publisher.

Published 2022 by Orange Blossom Publishing
Maitland, Florida
www.orangeblossombooks.com

ISBN: 978-1-949935-46-2

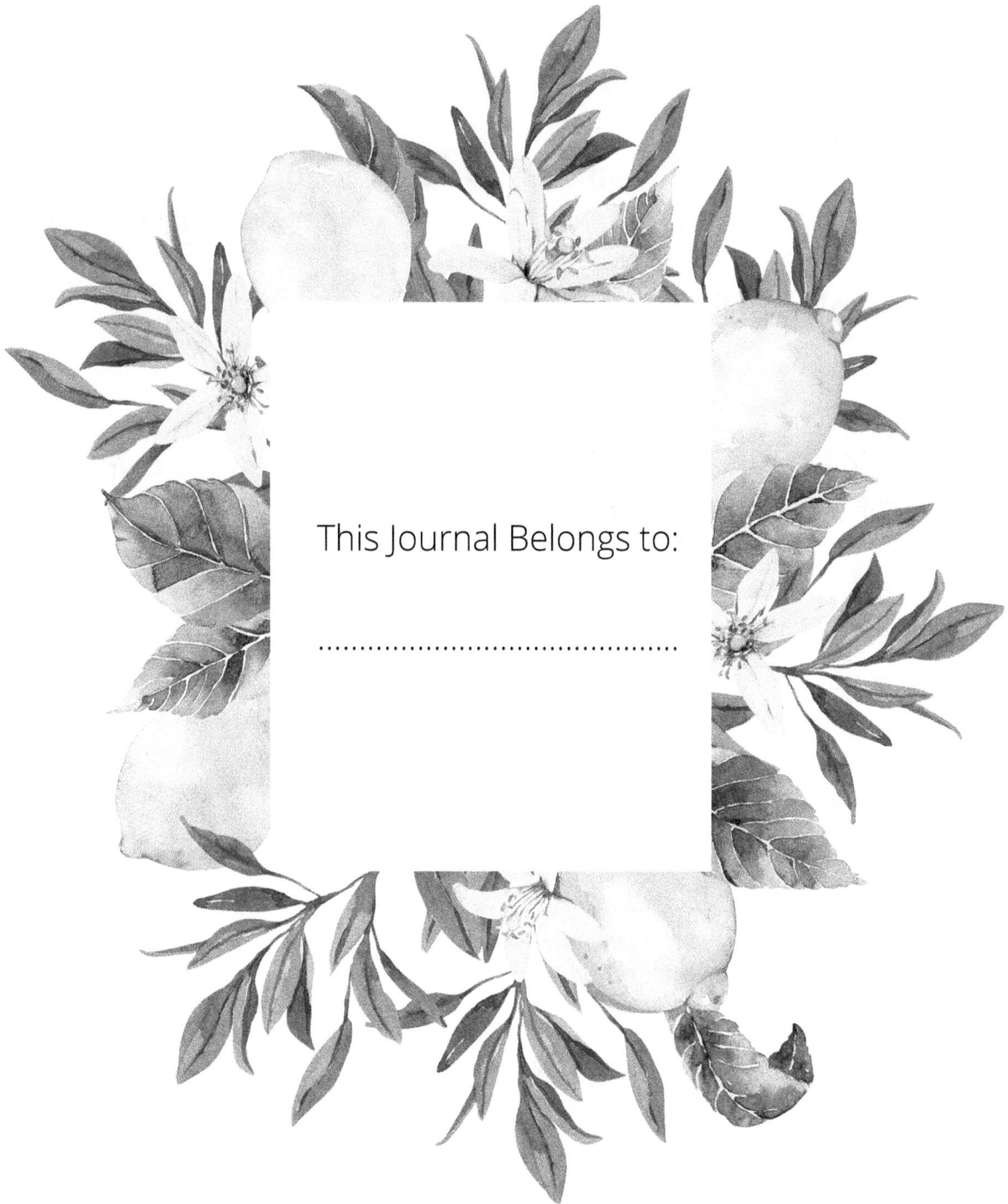

This Journal Belongs to:

....

"Acceptance doesn't mean resignation; it means
understanding that something is what it is and that
there's got to be a way through it."
- Michael J. Fox

A Note from Arielle

Crafting this journal has been very personal for me. I've suffered from chronic pain for many years due to a variety of medical conditions. Pain steals your time and happiness on bad days. And for those who have medical conditions, it's always around on the good days, too. Just hidden better in the background.

The National Library of Medicine states that "up to 85% of patients with chronic pain are affected by severe depression." Mayo Clinic explores the relationship between the two: "Sometimes pain and depression create a vicious cycle in which pain worsens symptoms of depression, and then the resulting depression worsens feelings of pain."

I've personally suffered from recurring depression since I was a teenager, and when chronic pain started taking center stage in my early thirties, my depression spiraled. I noticed a direct relationship with when I was feeling a lot of pain and the level of my depression. It seemed hopeless at times.

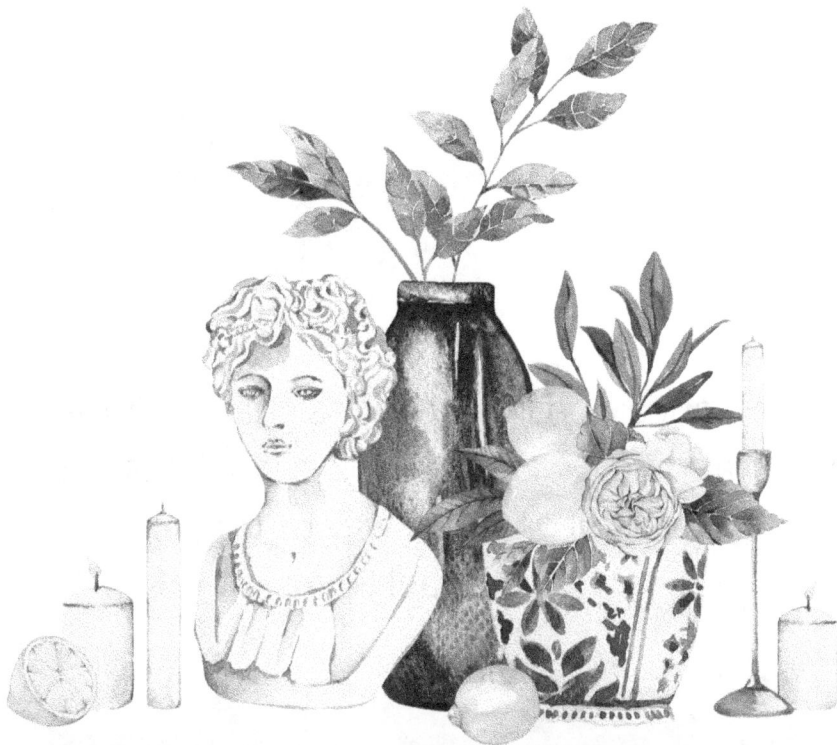

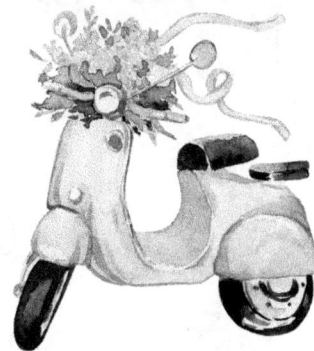

The first thing I want to say is that if your depression has gotten so bad, you feel like you can't live another day in pain, please get help. The biggest bright spot in my story came after my darkest period. I spent some time doing an intensive program with a mental health hospital to help me gain the mental tools I would need to make it through my hardest days.

Many of the strategies in this book came from my journey with mental health professionals who assisted me in getting a better mindset. Because I cannot stop the pain. That is a grim reality of chronic pain sufferers. We can do things to help prevent or treat the severity, but pain never fully disappears forever.

So what can we do?

Similarly to preventing and treating severe pain, we can take mitigating steps to help ease the depression that so often accompanies chronic pain. You'll find that different strategies work on different days. I've included a list to check options, so you can try out a variety of tools to help distract your mind and not spiral into those dark places. In the words of one of my wonderful therapists: "Action is the opposite of depression." You will need to DO to get through.

I hope you find this journal to be helpful in making you have brighter days, with more laughter and smiling. Even though we can't fully erase the pain, we can work toward having better days physically, and mentally. Most of all, I wish you serenity and that your days are filled with what every person is seeking, inner and outer calm.

Arielle

Opening Reflections

Take a moment to reflect on where you are now with your
mindset and pain, and where you'd like to be.

....

....

....

....

....

....

....

....

....

....

....

....

....

....

....

....

Opening Reflections

....

....

....

....

....

....

....

....

....

....

....

....

....

....

Quote Collector

Use this space to collect your favorite inspirational quotes

....

....

....

....

....

....

....

....

....

....

....

....

....

Quote Collector

Use this space to collect your favorite inspirational quotes

....

....

....

....

....

....

....

....

....

....

....

....

....

How To Use This Journal

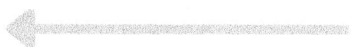

Monday........................ → Enter in the date

Sleep rating: 1 2 3 4 5 ← Score your night's sleep, 1 being the worst, 5 best

Mindset goal: ....
....

Eating goal: ....
....

Personal hygiene: bathe ...... teeth ......
style hair ...... get dressed ...... other ...... ← Make sure to do hygiene on your bad days, it's part of mental health!

Pain Management Strategies:
- [ ] deep breathing
- [ ] meditation
- [ ] visualization
- [ ] one object focus
- [ ] calming scents
- [ ] PMR
- [ ] rest
- [ ] music

Pain Management Strategy Explanations

Deep Breathing - Many women who've experienced labor and delivery can tell you the benefits of breathing through pain. Focus on deep, measured breaths in through the nose and out through the mouth during acute pain break throughs.

Visualization - This can be helpful when pain seems relentless and won't leave you alone. Close your eyes and picture a place where you feel completely comforted, the beach, your grandparents' house, wherever. Now focus on the sensory elements of this place. What do you see? Hear? Smell? Touch?

Calming Scents - Lavender is well known for its calming properties, so is bergamot. Try out different candles, essential oils, incense, or even dryer sheets to help provide aromatherapy.

How To Use This Journal

Rest - I have to confess, I put this one here for my own personal use. I try to make my body forge ahead, even when it's telling me no. Don't guilt yourself into being active when resting will help your body recuperate faster and better.

Meditation - It may be hard to focus your mind when it seems to be shouting the word "pain" over and over again, but spend some time researching types of meditation and see what's right for you. Then when the moment does come, you'll be ready.

One Object Focus - This is another great strategy for break-through acute pain. Pick out one object in the room and focus on it completely. Where did you get it? How do you think it was made? Who do you think made it? And so on...think everything you can about that one particular item.

PMR - This stands for progressive muscle relaxation. You start at the bottom of your body, clenching your toes and releasing and work all the way to the top. This is another strategy I recommend looking up in a search engine for more detailed information.

Music - Turn it up and jam out! Stick to upbeat, happy songs that make you sing along.

Something that made me smile:
....
....
Something I am proud of: ....
....
....
Something I am grateful for: ....
....
....
Something I am looking forward to: ....
....
....
Lowest pain level today: 1 2 3 4 5
Highest pain level today: 1 2 3 4 5

These quick daily reflections help keep you positive for the next day!

For these scales, 1 is little pain, 5 is high pain.

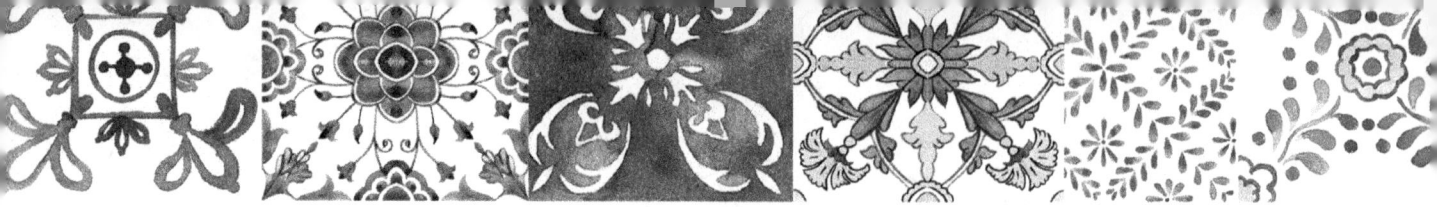

Week One

Goal for the week: ....
....

Days/Times I will leave the house or change settings: ....
....

When I will interact with friends or family: ....
....

Hobby I will work on: ....

Something new I'll try: ....

Medical tasks to do : ....
....
....

Monday..........................

Sleep rating: 1   2   3   4   5

Mindset goal: ....
....

Eating goal: ....
....

Personal hygiene: bathe ......   teeth ......
style hair ......   get dressed ......   other ......

Pain Management Strategies:

- [ ] deep breathing
- [ ] visualization
- [ ] calming scents
- [ ] rest
- [ ] meditation
- [ ] one object focus
- [ ] PMR
- [ ] music

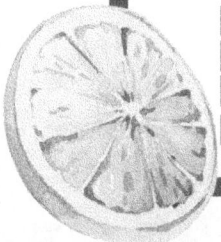

Something that made me smile:
....
....

Something I am proud of: ....
....

Something I am grateful for: ....
....
....

Something I am looking forward to: ....
....
....

Lowest pain level today: 1 2 3 4 5
Highest pain level today: 1 2 3 4 5

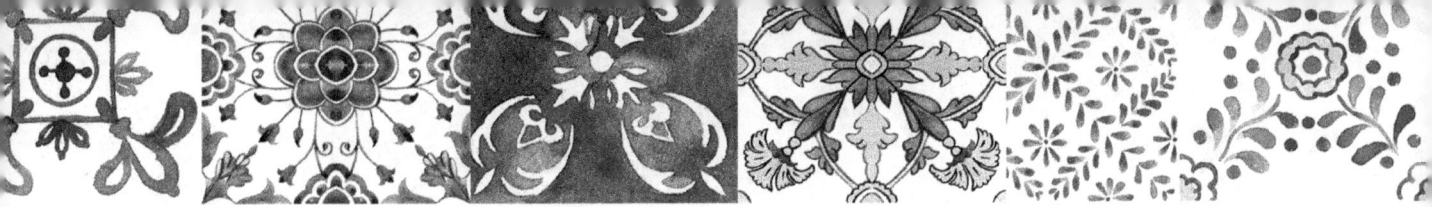

Week One

Tuesday.........................

Sleep rating: 1 2 3 4 5

Mindset goal: ....
....

Eating goal: ....
....

Personal hygiene: bathe ...... teeth ......
style hair ...... get dressed ...... other ......

Pain Management Strategies:

☐ deep breathing ☐ meditation
☐ visualization ☐ one object focus
☐ calming scents ☐ PMR
☐ rest ☐ music

Something that made me smile:
....
....

Something I am proud of: ....
....

Something I am grateful for: ....
....

Something I am looking forward to: ....
....
....

Lowest pain level today: 1 2 3 4 5
Highest pain level today: 1 2 3 4 5

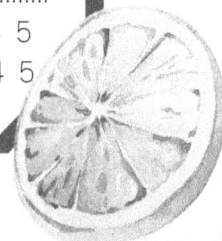

Wednesday.........................

Sleep rating: 1 2 3 4 5

Mindset goal: ....
....

Eating goal: ....
....

Personal hygiene: bathe ...... teeth ......
style hair ...... get dressed ...... other ......

Pain Management Strategies:

☐ deep breathing ☐ meditation
☐ visualization ☐ one object focus
☐ calming scents ☐ PMR
☐ rest ☐ music

Something that made me smile:
....
....

Something I am proud of: ....
....

Something I am grateful for: ....
....
....

Something I am looking forward to: ....
....
....

Lowest pain level today: 1 2 3 4 5
Highest pain level today: 1 2 3 4 5

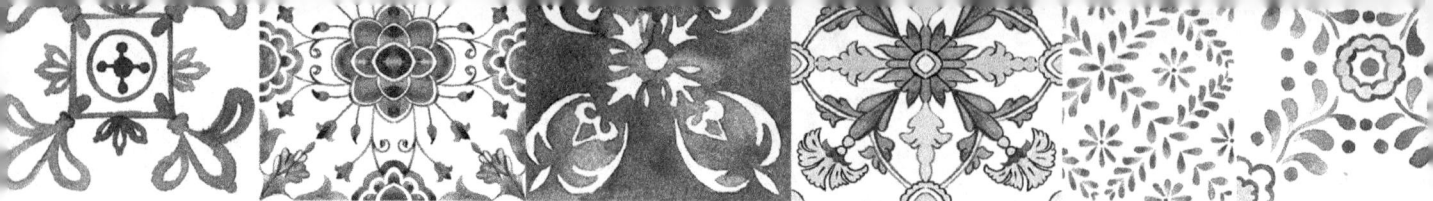

Week One

Thursday........................

Sleep rating: 1   2   3   4   5

Mindset goal: ....
....

Eating goal: ....
....

Personal hygiene: bathe ......   teeth ......
style hair ......   get dressed ......   other ......

Pain Management Strategies:

- [ ] deep breathing [ ] meditation
- [ ] visualization   [ ] one object focus
- [ ] calming scents [ ] PMR
- [ ] rest   [ ] music

Something that made me smile:
....
....

Something I am proud of: ....
....

Something I am grateful for: ....
....

Something I am looking forward to: ....
....
....

Lowest pain level today: 1   2   3   4   5
Highest pain level today: 1   2   3   4   5

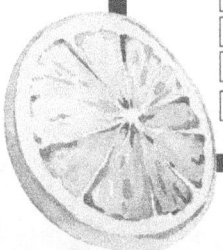

Friday..........................

Sleep rating: 1   2   3   4   5

Mindset goal: ....
....

Eating goal: ....
....

Personal hygiene: bathe ......   teeth ......
style hair ......   get dressed ......   other ......

Pain Management Strategies:

- [ ] deep breathing [ ] meditation
- [ ] visualization   [ ] one object focus
- [ ] calming scents [ ] PMR
- [ ] rest   [ ] music

Something that made me smile:
....
....

Something I am proud of: ....
....

Something I am grateful for: ....
....

Something I am looking forward to: ....
....
....

Lowest pain level today: 1   2   3   4   5
Highest pain level today: 1   2   3   4   5

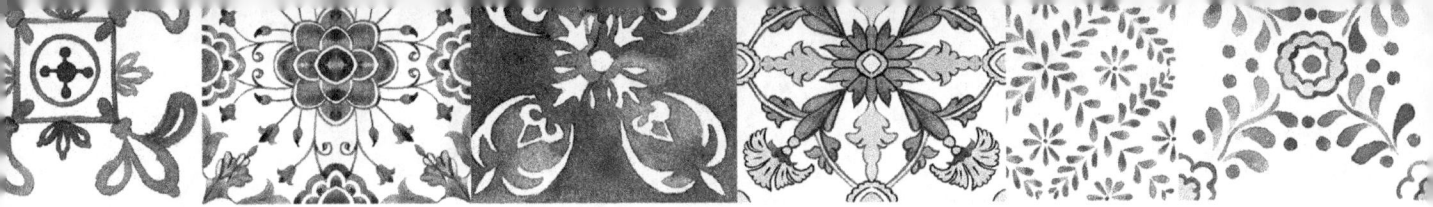

Week One

Saturday.......................

Sleep rating: 1 2 3 4 5

Mindset goal: ....
....

Eating goal: ....
....

Personal hygiene: bathe ...... teeth ......
style hair ...... get dressed ...... other ......

Pain Management Strategies:

☐ deep breathing ☐ meditation
☐ visualization ☐ one object focus
☐ calming scents ☐ PMR
☐ rest ☐ music

Something that made me smile:
....
....
Something I am proud of: ....
....
Something I am grateful for: ....
....
Something I am looking forward to: ....
....
....
Lowest pain level today: 1 2 3 4 5
Highest pain level today: 1 2 3 4 5

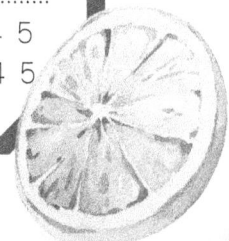

Sunday.........................

Sleep rating: 1 2 3 4 5

Mindset goal: ....
....

Eating goal: ....
....

Personal hygiene: bathe ...... teeth ......
style hair ...... get dressed ...... other ......

Pain Management Strategies:

☐ deep breathing ☐ meditation
☐ visualization ☐ one object focus
☐ calming scents ☐ PMR
☐ rest ☐ music

Something that made me smile:
....
....
Something I am proud of: ....
....
Something I am grateful for: ....
....
Something I am looking forward to: ....
....
....
Lowest pain level today: 1 2 3 4 5
Highest pain level today: 1 2 3 4 5

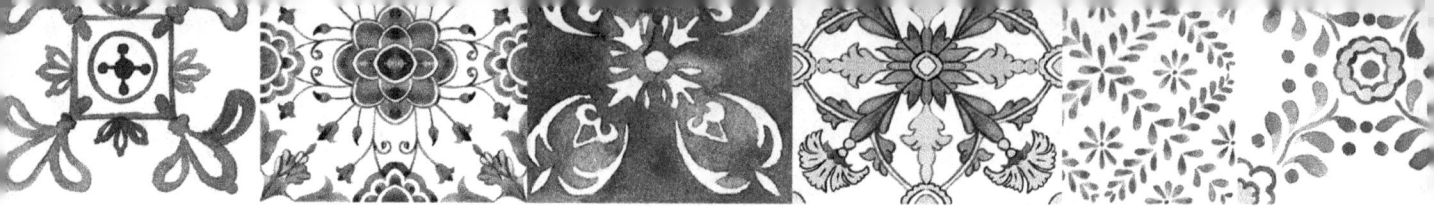

Week Two

Goal for the week: ....
....

Days/Times I will leave the house or change settings: ....
....

When I will interact with friends or family: ....
....

Hobby I will work on: ....

Something new I'll try: ....

Medical tasks to do : ....
....
....

Monday.........................

Sleep rating: 1   2   3   4   5

Mindset goal: ....
....

Eating goal: ....
....

Personal hygiene: bathe ......   teeth ......
style hair ......   get dressed ......   other ......

Pain Management Strategies:

☐ deep breathing ☐ meditation
☐ visualization   ☐ one object focus
☐ calming scents ☐ PMR
☐ rest   ☐ music

Something that made me smile:
....
....
Something I am proud of: ....
....
Something I am grateful for: ....
....
Something I am looking forward to: ....
....
....

Lowest pain level today: 1 2 3 4 5
Highest pain level today: 1 2 3 4 5

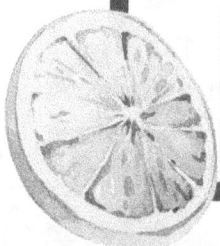

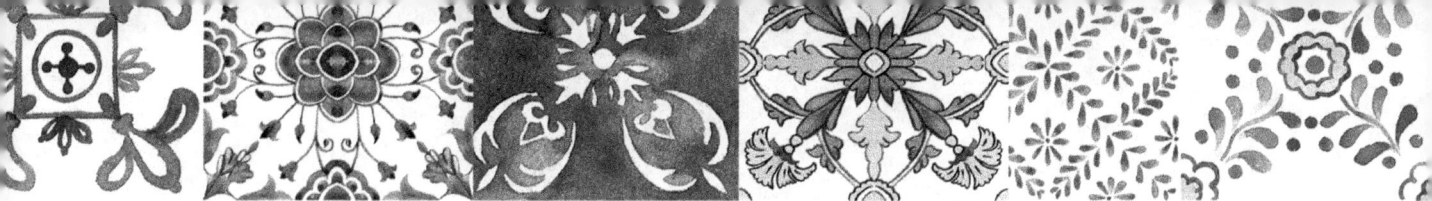

Tuesday.........................

Sleep rating: 1 2 3 4 5

Mindset goal: ....
....

Eating goal: ....
....

Personal hygiene: bathe ...... teeth ......
style hair ...... get dressed ...... other ......

Pain Management Strategies:

☐ deep breathing ☐ meditation
☐ visualization   ☐ one object focus
☐ calming scents ☐ PMR
☐ rest   ☐ music

Something that made me smile:
....
....

Something I am proud of: ....
....

Something I am grateful for: ....
....

Something I am looking forward to: ....
....

Lowest pain level today: 1 2 3 4 5
Highest pain level today: 1 2 3 4 5

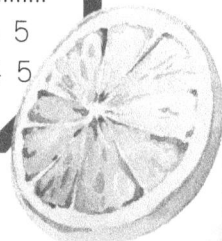

Wednesday.........................

Sleep rating: 1 2 3 4 5

Mindset goal: ....
....

Eating goal: ....
....

Personal hygiene: bathe ...... teeth ......
style hair ...... get dressed ...... other ......

Pain Management Strategies:

☐ deep breathing ☐ meditation
☐ visualization   ☐ one object focus
☐ calming scents ☐ PMR
☐ rest   ☐ music

Something that made me smile:
....
....

Something I am proud of: ....
....

Something I am grateful for: ....
....

Something I am looking forward to: ....
....

Lowest pain level today: 1 2 3 4 5
Highest pain level today: 1 2 3 4 5

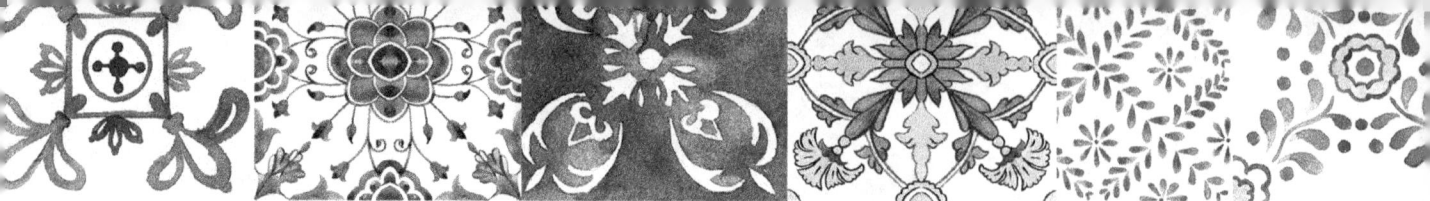

Thursday.....................

Sleep rating: 1 2 3 4 5

Mindset goal: ....
....

Eating goal: ....
....

Personal hygiene: bathe ...... teeth ......
style hair ...... get dressed ...... other ......

Pain Management Strategies:

☐ deep breathing ☐ meditation
☐ visualization ☐ one object focus
☐ calming scents ☐ PMR
☐ rest ☐ music

Something that made me smile:
....
....

Something I am proud of: ....
....

Something I am grateful for: ....
....

Something I am looking forward to: ....
....
....

Lowest pain level today: 1 2 3 4 5
Highest pain level today: 1 2 3 4 5

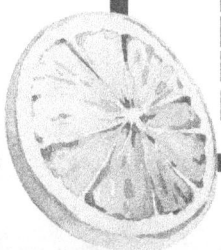

Friday........................

Sleep rating: 1 2 3 4 5

Mindset goal: ....
....

Eating goal: ....
....

Personal hygiene: bathe ...... teeth ......
style hair ...... get dressed ...... other ......

Pain Management Strategies:

☐ deep breathing ☐ meditation
☐ visualization ☐ one object focus
☐ calming scents ☐ PMR
☐ rest ☐ music

Something that made me smile:
....
....

Something I am proud of: ....
....

Something I am grateful for: ....
....

Something I am looking forward to: ....
....
....

Lowest pain level today: 1 2 3 4 5
Highest pain level today: 1 2 3 4 5

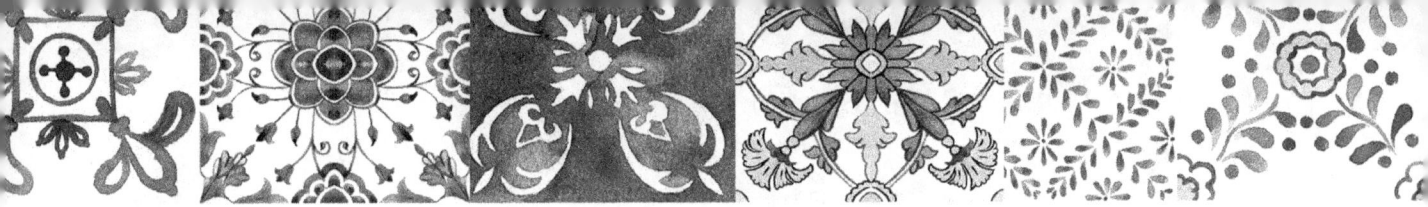

Saturday.......................

Sleep rating: 1 2 3 4 5

Mindset goal: ....

....

Eating goal: ....

....

Personal hygiene: bathe ......   teeth ......
style hair ......   get dressed ......   other ......

Pain Management Strategies:

☐ deep breathing ☐ meditation
☐ visualization ☐ one object focus
☐ calming scents ☐ PMR
☐ rest ☐ music

Something that made me smile:
....
....
Something I am proud of: ....
....
Something I am grateful for: ....
....
Something I am looking forward to: ....
....
....

Lowest pain level today: 1 2 3 4 5
Highest pain level today: 1 2 3 4 5

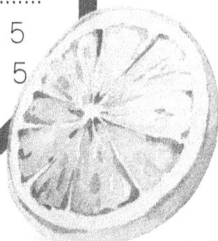

Sunday..........................

Sleep rating: 1 2 3 4 5

Mindset goal: ....

....

Eating goal: ....

....

Personal hygiene: bathe ......   teeth ......
style hair ......   get dressed ......   other ......

Pain Management Strategies:

☐ deep breathing ☐ meditation
☐ visualization ☐ one object focus
☐ calming scents ☐ PMR
☐ rest ☐ music

Something that made me smile:
....
....
Something I am proud of: ....
....
Something I am grateful for: ....
....
....
Something I am looking forward to: ....
....
....

Lowest pain level today: 1 2 3 4 5
Highest pain level today: 1 2 3 4 5

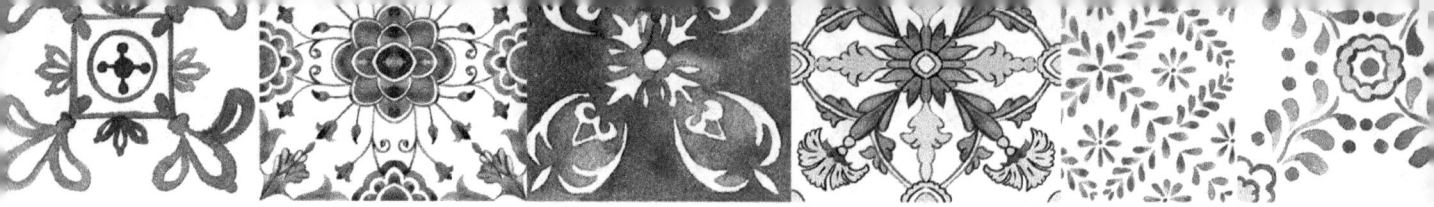

Week Three

Goal for the week: ....
....

Days/Times I will leave the house or change settings: ....
....

When I will interact with friends or family: ....
....

Hobby I will work on: ....

Something new I'll try: ....

Medical tasks to do : ....
....
....

Monday..........................

Sleep rating: 1   2   3   4   5

Mindset goal: ....
....

Eating goal: ....
....

Personal hygiene: bathe ......   teeth ......
style hair ......   get dressed ......   other ......

Pain Management Strategies:

- [ ] deep breathing
- [ ] visualization
- [ ] calming scents
- [ ] rest
- [ ] meditation
- [ ] one object focus
- [ ] PMR
- [ ] music

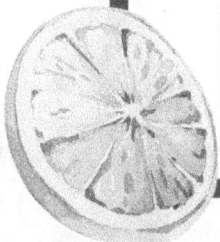

Something that made me smile:
....
....

Something I am proud of: ....
....

Something I am grateful for: ....
....
....

Something I am looking forward to: ....
....
....

Lowest pain level today: 1 2 3 4 5
Highest pain level today: 1 2 3 4 5

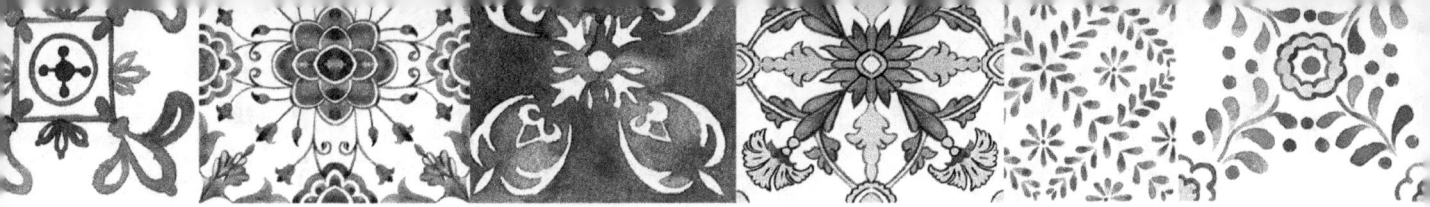

Week Three

Tuesday........................

Sleep rating: 1 2 3 4 5

Mindset goal: ....
....

Eating goal: ....
....

Personal hygiene: bathe ......   teeth ......
style hair ......   get dressed ......   other ......

Pain Management Strategies:

☐ deep breathing ☐ meditation
☐ visualization ☐ one object focus
☐ calming scents ☐ PMR
☐ rest ☐ music

Something that made me smile:
....
....
Something I am proud of: ....
....
Something I am grateful for: ....
....
Something I am looking forward to: ....
....
....
Lowest pain level today: 1 2 3 4 5
Highest pain level today: 1 2 3 4 5

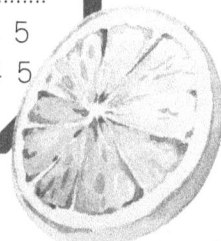

Wednesday........................

Sleep rating: 1 2 3 4 5

Mindset goal: ....
....

Eating goal: ....
....

Personal hygiene: bathe ......   teeth ......
style hair ......   get dressed ......   other ......

Pain Management Strategies:

☐ deep breathing ☐ meditation
☐ visualization ☐ one object focus
☐ calming scents ☐ PMR
☐ rest ☐ music

Something that made me smile:
....
....
Something I am proud of: ....
....
Something I am grateful for: ....
....
Something I am looking forward to: ....
....
....
Lowest pain level today: 1 2 3 4 5
Highest pain level today: 1 2 3 4 5

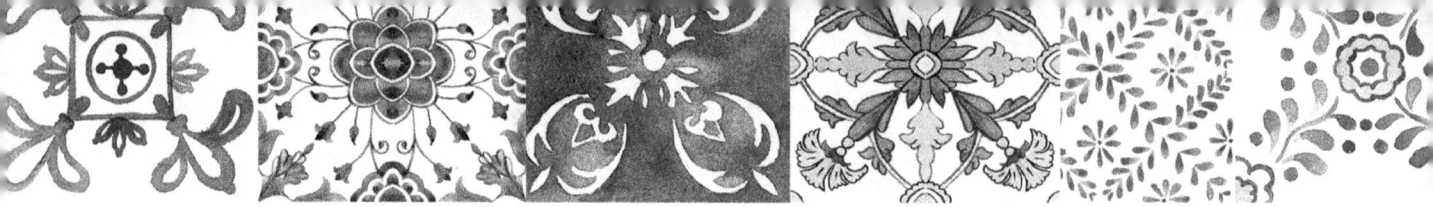

Thursday.....................

Sleep rating: 1 2 3 4 5

Mindset goal: ....
....

Eating goal: ....
....

Personal hygiene: bathe ...... teeth ......
style hair ...... get dressed ...... other ......

Pain Management Strategies:

☐ deep breathing ☐ meditation
☐ visualization ☐ one object focus
☐ calming scents ☐ PMR
☐ rest ☐ music

Something that made me smile:
....
....

Something I am proud of: ....

Something I am grateful for: ....

Something I am looking forward to: ....

Lowest pain level today: 1 2 3 4 5
Highest pain level today: 1 2 3 4 5

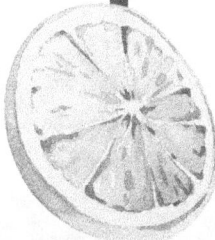

Friday........................

Sleep rating: 1 2 3 4 5

Mindset goal: ....
....

Eating goal: ....
....

Personal hygiene: bathe ...... teeth ......
style hair ...... get dressed ...... other ......

Pain Management Strategies:

☐ deep breathing ☐ meditation
☐ visualization ☐ one object focus
☐ calming scents ☐ PMR
☐ rest ☐ music

Something that made me smile:
....
....

Something I am proud of: ....

Something I am grateful for: ....

Something I am looking forward to: ....

Lowest pain level today: 1 2 3 4 5
Highest pain level today: 1 2 3 4 5

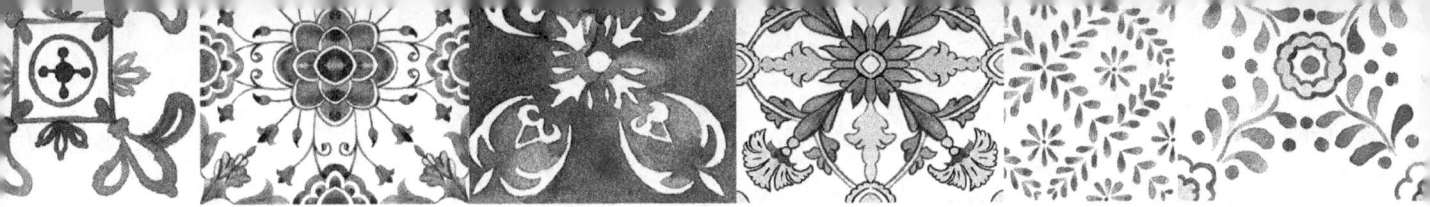

Week Three

Saturday........................

Sleep rating: 1 2 3 4 5

Mindset goal: ....
....

Eating goal: ....
....

Personal hygiene: bathe ......   teeth ......
style hair ......   get dressed ......   other ......

Pain Management Strategies:

☐ deep breathing   ☐ meditation
☐ visualization   ☐ one object focus
☐ calming scents   ☐ PMR
☐ rest   ☐ music

Something that made me smile:
....
....
Something I am proud of: ....
....
Something I am grateful for: ....
....
Something I am looking forward to: ....
....
....
Lowest pain level today: 1 2 3 4 5
Highest pain level today: 1 2 3 4 5

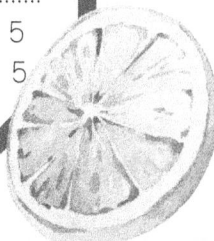

Sunday........................

Sleep rating: 1 2 3 4 5

Mindset goal: ....
....

Eating goal: ....
....

Personal hygiene: bathe ......   teeth ......
style hair ......   get dressed ......   other ......

Pain Management Strategies:

☐ deep breathing   ☐ meditation
☐ visualization   ☐ one object focus
☐ calming scents   ☐ PMR
☐ rest   ☐ music

Something that made me smile:
....
....
Something I am proud of: ....
....
Something I am grateful for: ....
....
....
Something I am looking forward to: ....
....
....
Lowest pain level today: 1 2 3 4 5
Highest pain level today: 1 2 3 4 5

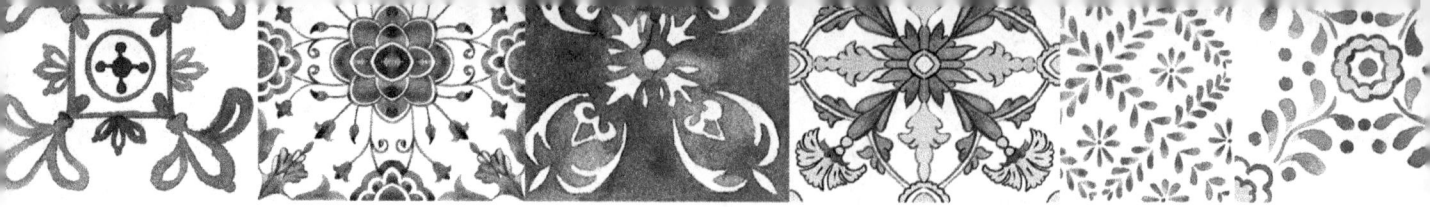

Week Four

Goal for the week: ....

....

Days/Times I will leave the house or change settings: ....

....

When I will interact with friends or family: ....

....

Hobby I will work on: ....

Something new I'll try: ....

Medical tasks to do : ....

....

....

Monday.........................

Sleep rating: 1 2 3 4 5

Mindset goal: ....

....

Eating goal: ....

....

Personal hygiene: bathe ......   teeth ......
style hair ......   get dressed ......   other ......

Pain Management Strategies:

☐ deep breathing ☐ meditation
☐ visualization ☐ one object focus
☐ calming scents ☐ PMR
☐ rest ☐ music

Something that made me smile:

....

....

Something I am proud of: ....

....

Something I am grateful for: ....

....

....

Something I am looking forward to: ....

....

....

Lowest pain level today: 1 2 3 4 5
Highest pain level today: 1 2 3 4 5

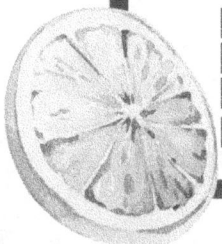

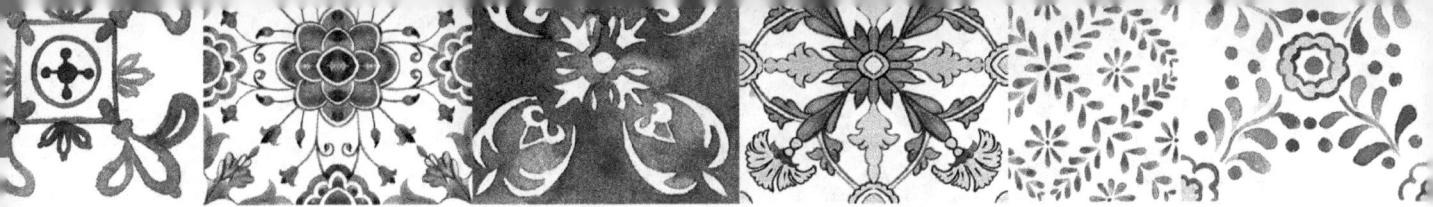

Tuesday..........................

Sleep rating: 1 2 3 4 5

Mindset goal: ....
....

Eating goal: ....
....

Personal hygiene: bathe ......   teeth ......
style hair ......   get dressed ......   other ......

Pain Management Strategies:

☐ deep breathing ☐ meditation
☐ visualization ☐ one object focus
☐ calming scents ☐ PMR
☐ rest ☐ music

Something that made me smile:
....
....
Something I am proud of: ....
....
Something I am grateful for: ....
....
Something I am looking forward to: ....
....
....
Lowest pain level today: 1 2 3 4 5
Highest pain level today: 1 2 3 4 5

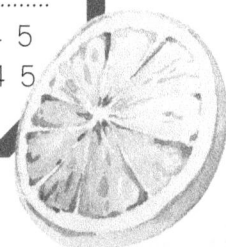

Wednesday...........................

Sleep rating: 1 2 3 4 5

Mindset goal: ....
....

Eating goal: ....
....

Personal hygiene: bathe ......   teeth ......
style hair ......   get dressed ......   other ......

Pain Management Strategies:

☐ deep breathing ☐ meditation
☐ visualization ☐ one object focus
☐ calming scents ☐ PMR
☐ rest ☐ music

Something that made me smile:
....
....
Something I am proud of: ....
....
....
Something I am grateful for: ....
....
Something I am looking forward to: ....
....
....
Lowest pain level today: 1 2 3 4 5
Highest pain level today: 1 2 3 4 5

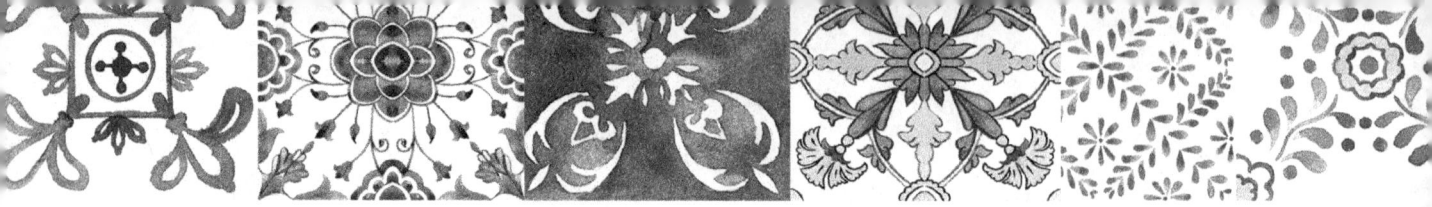

Thursday.....................

Sleep rating: 1 2 3 4 5

Mindset goal: ....
....

Eating goal: ....
....

Personal hygiene: bathe ......   teeth ......
style hair ......   get dressed ......   other ......

Pain Management Strategies:

☐ deep breathing ☐ meditation
☐ visualization   ☐ one object focus
☐ calming scents ☐ PMR
☐ rest   ☐ music

Something that made me smile:
....
....
Something I am proud of: ....
....
Something I am grateful for: ....
....
Something I am looking forward to: ....
....
....
Lowest pain level today: 1 2 3 4 5
Highest pain level today: 1 2 3 4 5

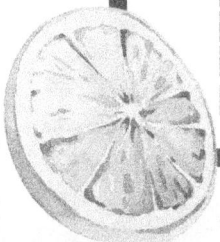

Friday.........................

Sleep rating: 1 2 3 4 5

Mindset goal: ....
....

Eating goal: ....
....

Personal hygiene: bathe ......   teeth ......
style hair ......   get dressed ......   other ......

Pain Management Strategies:

☐ deep breathing ☐ meditation
☐ visualization   ☐ one object focus
☐ calming scents ☐ PMR
☐ rest   ☐ music

Something that made me smile:
....
....
Something I am proud of: ....
....
Something I am grateful for: ....
....
Something I am looking forward to: ....
....
....
Lowest pain level today: 1 2 3 4 5
Highest pain level today: 1 2 3 4 5

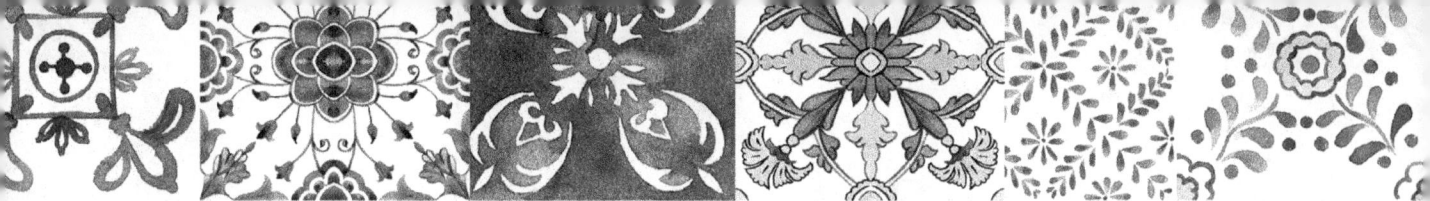

Week Four

Saturday.......................

Sleep rating: 1 2 3 4 5

Mindset goal: ....
....

Eating goal: ....
....

Personal hygiene: bathe ...... teeth ......
style hair ...... get dressed ...... other ......

Pain Management Strategies:

- ☐ deep breathing ☐ meditation
- ☐ visualization ☐ one object focus
- ☐ calming scents ☐ PMR
- ☐ rest ☐ music

Something that made me smile:
....
....
Something I am proud of: ....
....
Something I am grateful for: ....
....
Something I am looking forward to: ....
....

Lowest pain level today: 1 2 3 4 5
Highest pain level today: 1 2 3 4 5

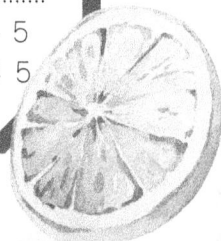

Sunday........................

Sleep rating: 1 2 3 4 5

Mindset goal: ....
....

Eating goal: ....
....

Personal hygiene: bathe ...... teeth ......
style hair ...... get dressed ...... other ......

Pain Management Strategies:

- ☐ deep breathing ☐ meditation
- ☐ visualization ☐ one object focus
- ☐ calming scents ☐ PMR
- ☐ rest ☐ music

Something that made me smile:
....
....
Something I am proud of: ....
....
Something I am grateful for: ....
....
Something I am looking forward to: ....
....

Lowest pain level today: 1 2 3 4 5
Highest pain level today: 1 2 3 4 5

Monthly Reflection

Think about how your mental health was this month. Did you use the strategies? When were you your best? Your worst?

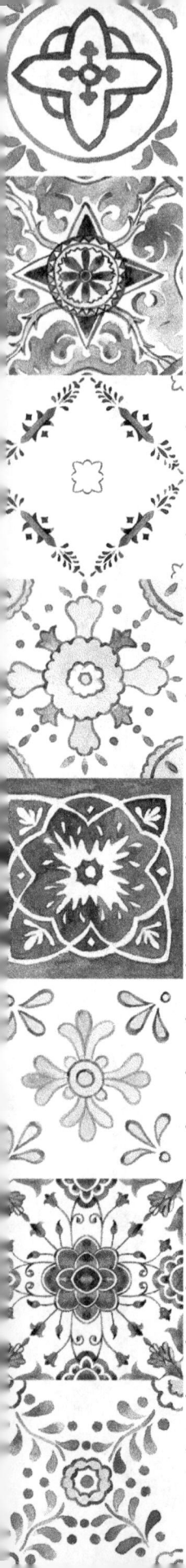

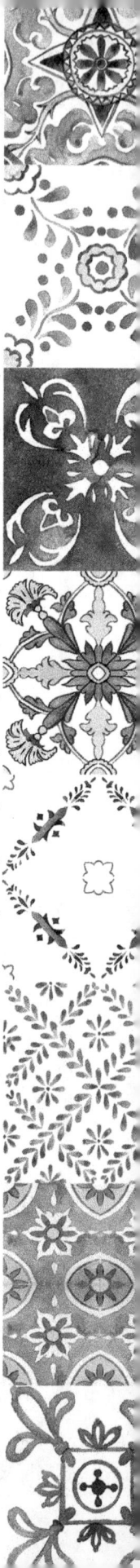

....
....
....
....
....
....
....
....
....
....
....
....
....
....
....
....
....

Happy Distraction

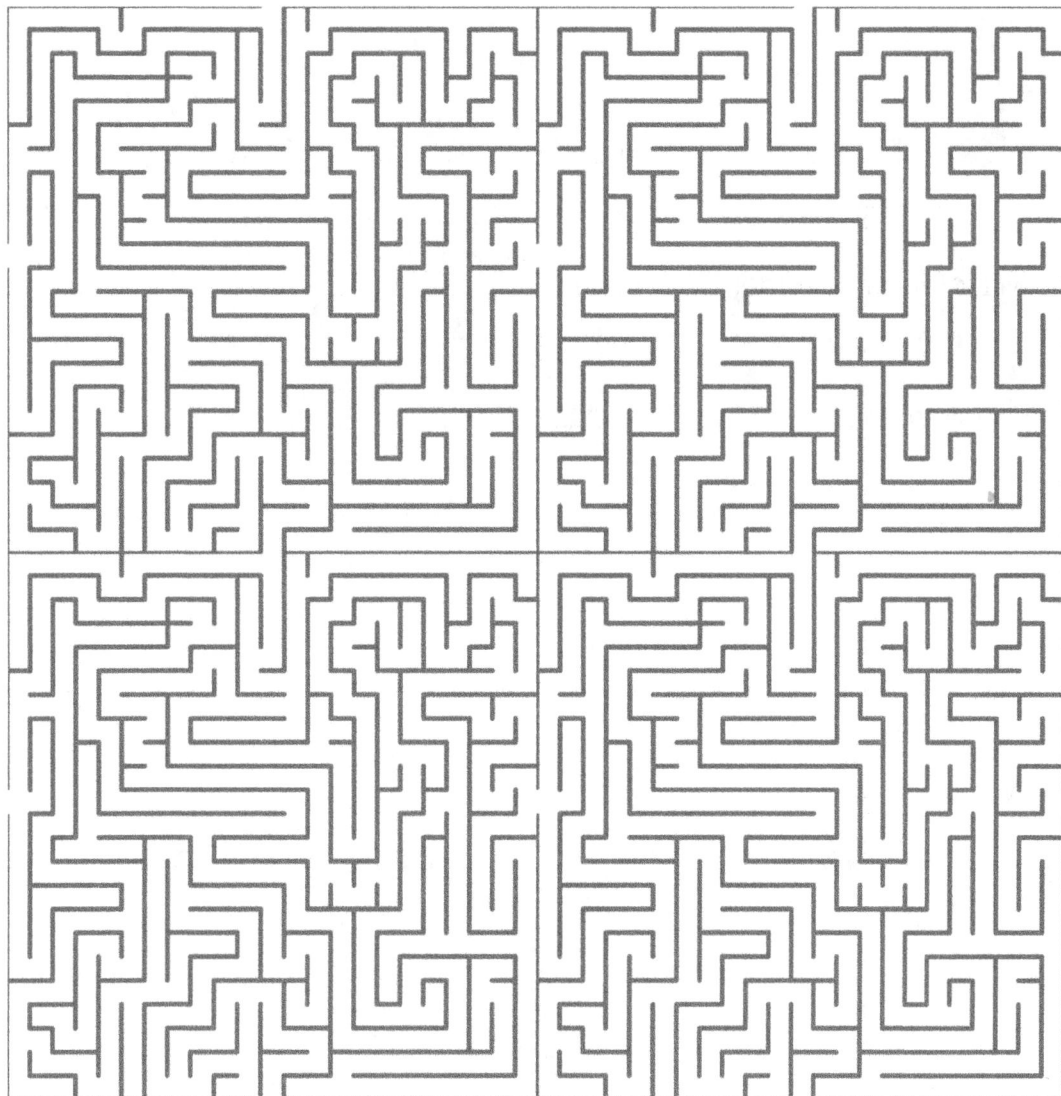

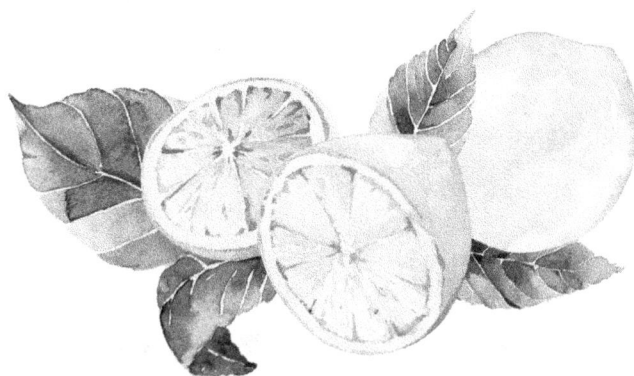

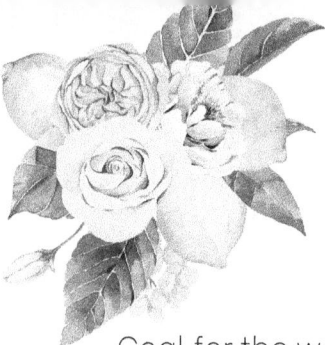

Week Five

Goal for the week: ....
....

Days/Times I will leave the house or change settings: ....
....

When I will interact with friends or family: ....
....

Hobby I will work on: ....

Something new I'll try: ....

Medical tasks to do : ....
....
....

Monday.........................

Sleep rating: 1   2   3   4   5

Mindset goal: ....
....

Eating goal: ....
....

Personal hygiene: bathe ......   teeth ......
style hair ......   get dressed ......   other ......

Pain Management Strategies:

- [ ] deep breathing [ ] meditation
- [ ] visualization [ ] one object focus
- [ ] calming scents [ ] PMR
- [ ] rest [ ] music

Something that made me smile:
....
....

Something I am proud of: ....
....

Something I am grateful for: ....
....

Something I am looking forward to: ....
....
....

Lowest pain level today: 1 2 3 4 5
Highest pain level today: 1 2 3 4 5

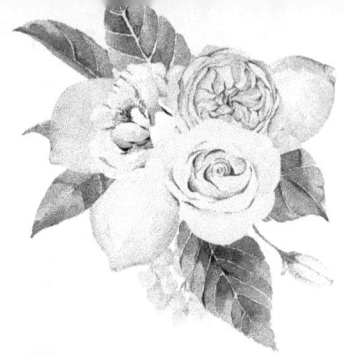

Week Five

Tuesday...................

Sleep rating: 1 2 3 4 5

Mindset goal: ....
....

Eating goal: ....
....

Personal hygiene: bathe ...... teeth ......
style hair ...... get dressed ...... other ......

Pain Management Strategies:

☐ deep breathing ☐ meditation
☐ visualization ☐ one object focus
☐ calming scents ☐ PMR
☐ rest ☐ music

Something that made me smile:
....
....
Something I am proud of: ....
....
Something I am grateful for: ....
....
....
Something I am looking forward to: ....
....
....

Lowest pain level today: 1 2 3 4 5
Highest pain level today: 1 2 3 4 5

Wednesday.........................

Sleep rating: 1 2 3 4 5

Mindset goal: ....
....

Eating goal: ....
....

Personal hygiene: bathe ...... teeth ......
style hair ...... get dressed ...... other ......

Pain Management Strategies:

☐ deep breathing ☐ meditation
☐ visualization ☐ one object focus
☐ calming scents ☐ PMR
☐ rest ☐ music

Something that made me smile:
....
....
Something I am proud of: ....
....
Something I am grateful for: ....
....
....
Something I am looking forward to: ....
....
....

Lowest pain level today: 1 2 3 4 5
Highest pain level today: 1 2 3 4 5

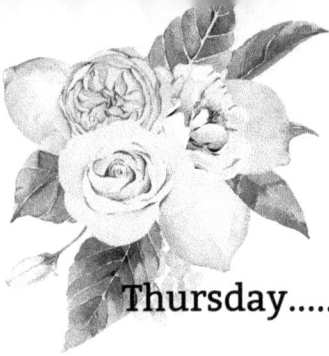

Sleep rating: 1 2 3 4 5

Mindset goal: ....
....

Eating goal: ....
....

Personal hygiene: bathe ......   teeth ......
style hair ......   get dressed ......   other ......

Pain Management Strategies:

☐ deep breathing   ☐ meditation
☐ visualization   ☐ one object focus
☐ calming scents   ☐ PMR
☐ rest   ☐ music

Something that made me smile:
....
....
Something I am proud of: ....
....
Something I am grateful for: ....
....
Something I am looking forward to: ....
....
....

Lowest pain level today: 1 2 3 4 5
Highest pain level today: 1 2 3 4 5

Friday.........................

Sleep rating: 1 2 3 4 5

Mindset goal: ....
....

Eating goal: ....
....

Personal hygiene: bathe ......   teeth ......
style hair ......   get dressed ......   other ......

Pain Management Strategies:

☐ deep breathing   ☐ meditation
☐ visualization   ☐ one object focus
☐ calming scents   ☐ PMR
☐ rest   ☐ music

Something that made me smile:
....
....
Something I am proud of: ....
....
Something I am grateful for: ....
....
....
Something I am looking forward to: ....
....

Lowest pain level today: 1 2 3 4 5
Highest pain level today: 1 2 3 4 5

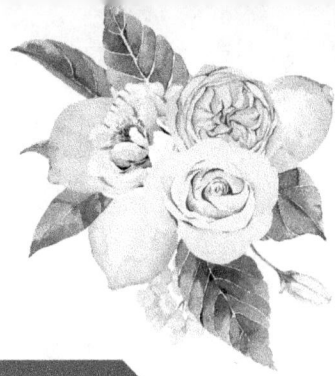

Saturday.....................

Sleep rating: 1 2 3 4 5

Mindset goal: ....
....

Eating goal: ....
....

Personal hygiene: bathe ...... teeth ......
style hair ...... get dressed ...... other ......

Pain Management Strategies:

☐ deep breathing ☐ meditation
☐ visualization ☐ one object focus
☐ calming scents ☐ PMR
☐ rest ☐ music

Something that made me smile:
....
....
Something I am proud of: ....
....
Something I am grateful for: ....
....
....
Something I am looking forward to: ....
....
....

Lowest pain level today: 1 2 3 4 5
Highest pain level today: 1 2 3 4 5

Sunday.........................

Sleep rating: 1 2 3 4 5

Mindset goal: ....
....

Eating goal: ....
....

Personal hygiene: bathe ...... teeth ......
style hair ...... get dressed ...... other ......

Pain Management Strategies:

☐ deep breathing ☐ meditation
☐ visualization ☐ one object focus
☐ calming scents ☐ PMR
☐ rest ☐ music

Something that made me smile:
....
....
Something I am proud of: ....
....
Something I am grateful for: ....
....
....
Something I am looking forward to: ....
....
....

Lowest pain level today: 1 2 3 4 5
Highest pain level today: 1 2 3 4 5

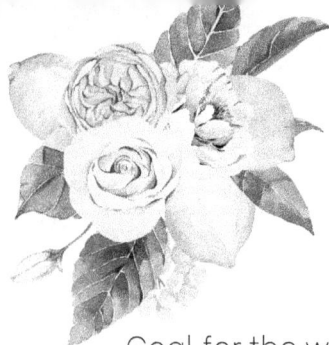

Week Six

Goal for the week: ....
....

Days/Times I will leave the house or change settings: ....
....

When I will interact with friends or family: ....
....

Hobby I will work on: ....

Something new I'll try: ....

Medical tasks to do : ....
....
....

Monday.........................

Sleep rating: 1 2 3 4 5

Mindset goal: ....
....

Eating goal: ....
....

Personal hygiene: bathe ......   teeth ......
style hair ......   get dressed ......   other ......

Pain Management Strategies:

- [ ] deep breathing
- [ ] visualization
- [ ] calming scents
- [ ] rest
- [ ] meditation
- [ ] one object focus
- [ ] PMR
- [ ] music

Something that made me smile:
....
....
Something I am proud of: ....
....
....
Something I am grateful for: ....
....
....
Something I am looking forward to: ....
....
....

Lowest pain level today: 1 2 3 4 5
Highest pain level today: 1 2 3 4 5

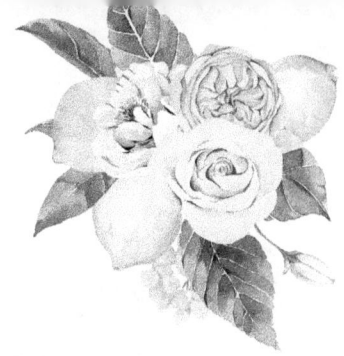

Week Six

Tuesday..........................

Sleep rating: 1 2 3 4 5

Mindset goal: ....
....

Eating goal: ....
....

Personal hygiene: bathe ...... teeth ......
style hair ...... get dressed ...... other ......

Pain Management Strategies:

☐ deep breathing ☐ meditation
☐ visualization ☐ one object focus
☐ calming scents ☐ PMR
☐ rest ☐ music

Something that made me smile:
....
....
Something I am proud of: ....
....
....
Something I am grateful for: ....
....
....
Something I am looking forward to: ....
....
....

Lowest pain level today: 1 2 3 4 5
Highest pain level today: 1 2 3 4 5

Wednesday..........................

Sleep rating: 1 2 3 4 5

Mindset goal: ....
....

Eating goal: ....
....

Personal hygiene: bathe ...... teeth ......
style hair ...... get dressed ...... other ......

Pain Management Strategies:

☐ deep breathing ☐ meditation
☐ visualization ☐ one object focus
☐ calming scents ☐ PMR
☐ rest ☐ music

Something that made me smile:
....
....
Something I am proud of: ....
....
....
Something I am grateful for: ....
....
....
Something I am looking forward to: ....
....
....

Lowest pain level today: 1 2 3 4 5
Highest pain level today: 1 2 3 4 5

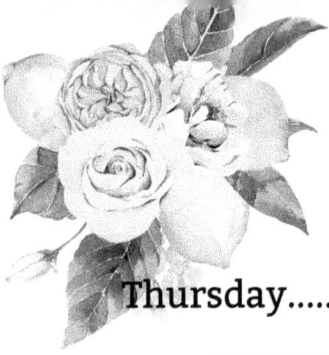

Thursday..................... *Week Six*

Sleep rating: 1 2 3 4 5

Mindset goal: ....
....

Eating goal: ....
....

Personal hygiene: bathe ...... teeth ......
style hair ...... get dressed ...... other ......

Pain Management Strategies:

☐ deep breathing ☐ meditation
☐ visualization ☐ one object focus
☐ calming scents ☐ PMR
☐ rest ☐ music

Something that made me smile:
....
....
Something I am proud of: ....
....
....
Something I am grateful for: ....
....
....
Something I am looking forward to: ....
....
....
Lowest pain level today: 1 2 3 4 5
Highest pain level today: 1 2 3 4 5

Friday.........................

Sleep rating: 1 2 3 4 5

Mindset goal: ....
....

Eating goal: ....
....

Personal hygiene: bathe ...... teeth ......
style hair ...... get dressed ...... other ......

Pain Management Strategies:

☐ deep breathing ☐ meditation
☐ visualization ☐ one object focus
☐ calming scents ☐ PMR
☐ rest ☐ music

Something that made me smile:
....
....
Something I am proud of: ....
....
....
Something I am grateful for: ....
....
....
Something I am looking forward to: ....
....
....
Lowest pain level today: 1 2 3 4 5
Highest pain level today: 1 2 3 4 5

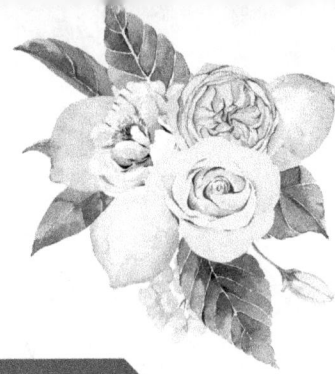

Week Six

Saturday.......................

Sleep rating: 1 2 3 4 5

Mindset goal: ....
....

Eating goal: ....
....

Personal hygiene: bathe ...... teeth ......
style hair ...... get dressed ...... other ......

Pain Management Strategies:

☐ deep breathing ☐ meditation
☐ visualization ☐ one object focus
☐ calming scents ☐ PMR
☐ rest ☐ music

Something that made me smile:
....
....
Something I am proud of: ....
....
Something I am grateful for: ....
....
....
Something I am looking forward to: ....
....
....

Lowest pain level today: 1 2 3 4 5
Highest pain level today: 1 2 3 4 5

Sunday.........................

Sleep rating: 1 2 3 4 5

Mindset goal: ....
....

Eating goal: ....
....

Personal hygiene: bathe ...... teeth ......
style hair ...... get dressed ...... other ......

Pain Management Strategies:

☐ deep breathing ☐ meditation
☐ visualization ☐ one object focus
☐ calming scents ☐ PMR
☐ rest ☐ music

Something that made me smile:
....
....
Something I am proud of: ....
....
Something I am grateful for: ....
....
....
Something I am looking forward to: ....
....
....

Lowest pain level today: 1 2 3 4 5
Highest pain level today: 1 2 3 4 5

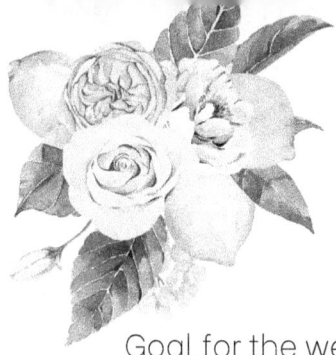

Week Seven

Goal for the week: ....
....

Days/Times I will leave the house or change settings: ....
....

When I will interact with friends or family: ....
....

Hobby I will work on: ....

Something new I'll try: ....

Medical tasks to do : ....
....
....

Monday........................

Sleep rating: 1 2 3 4 5

Mindset goal: ....
....

Eating goal: ....
....

Personal hygiene: bathe ......   teeth ......
style hair ......   get dressed ......   other ......

Pain Management Strategies:

☐ deep breathing ☐ meditation
☐ visualization ☐ one object focus
☐ calming scents ☐ PMR
☐ rest ☐ music

Something that made me smile:
....
....

Something I am proud of: ....
....

Something I am grateful for: ....
....
....

Something I am looking forward to: ....
....
....

Lowest pain level today: 1 2 3 4 5
Highest pain level today: 1 2 3 4 5

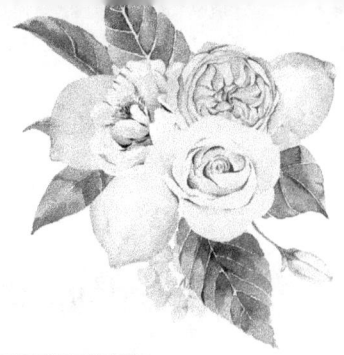

Week Seven

Tuesday........................

Sleep rating: 1 2 3 4 5

Mindset goal: ....
....

Eating goal: ....
....

Personal hygiene: bathe ...... teeth ......
style hair ...... get dressed ...... other ......

Pain Management Strategies:

☐ deep breathing ☐ meditation
☐ visualization ☐ one object focus
☐ calming scents ☐ PMR
☐ rest ☐ music

Something that made me smile:
....
....

Something I am proud of: ....
....

Something I am grateful for: ....
....

Something I am looking forward to: ....
....

Lowest pain level today: 1 2 3 4 5
Highest pain level today: 1 2 3 4 5

Wednesday........................

Sleep rating: 1 2 3 4 5

Mindset goal: ....
....

Eating goal: ....
....

Personal hygiene: bathe ...... teeth ......
style hair ...... get dressed ...... other ......

Pain Management Strategies:

☐ deep breathing ☐ meditation
☐ visualization ☐ one object focus
☐ calming scents ☐ PMR
☐ rest ☐ music

Something that made me smile:
....
....

Something I am proud of: ....
....

Something I am grateful for: ....
....

Something I am looking forward to: ....
....

Lowest pain level today: 1 2 3 4 5
Highest pain level today: 1 2 3 4 5

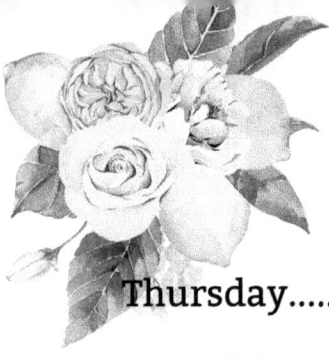

Thursday.....................

Sleep rating: 1 2 3 4 5

Mindset goal: ....
....

Eating goal: ....
....

Personal hygiene: bathe ......   teeth ......
style hair ......   get dressed ......   other ......

Pain Management Strategies:

- ☐ deep breathing   ☐ meditation
- ☐ visualization   ☐ one object focus
- ☐ calming scents   ☐ PMR
- ☐ rest   ☐ music

Something that made me smile:
....
....

Something I am proud of: ....

Something I am grateful for: ....

Something I am looking forward to: ....
....
....

Lowest pain level today: 1 2 3 4 5
Highest pain level today: 1 2 3 4 5

Friday.........................

Sleep rating: 1 2 3 4 5

Mindset goal: ....
....

Eating goal: ....
....

Personal hygiene: bathe ......   teeth ......
style hair ......   get dressed ......   other ......

Pain Management Strategies:

- ☐ deep breathing   ☐ meditation
- ☐ visualization   ☐ one object focus
- ☐ calming scents   ☐ PMR
- ☐ rest   ☐ music

Something that made me smile:
....
....

Something I am proud of: ....

Something I am grateful for: ....

Something I am looking forward to: ....
....
....

Lowest pain level today: 1 2 3 4 5
Highest pain level today: 1 2 3 4 5

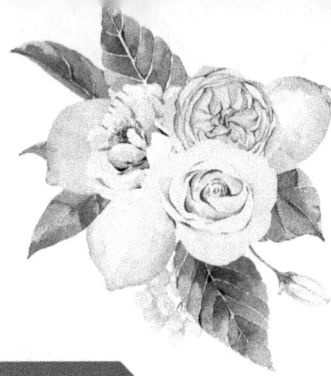

Week Seven

Saturday......................

Sleep rating: 1 2 3 4 5

Mindset goal: ....
....

Eating goal: ....
....

Personal hygiene: bathe ......   teeth ......
style hair ......   get dressed ......   other ......

Pain Management Strategies:

☐ deep breathing ☐ meditation
☐ visualization ☐ one object focus
☐ calming scents ☐ PMR
☐ rest ☐ music

Something that made me smile:
....
....
Something I am proud of: ....
....
Something I am grateful for: ....
....
....
Something I am looking forward to: ....
....
....
Lowest pain level today: 1 2 3 4 5
Highest pain level today: 1 2 3 4 5

Sunday.........................

Sleep rating: 1 2 3 4 5

Mindset goal: ....
....

Eating goal: ....
....

Personal hygiene: bathe ......   teeth ......
style hair ......   get dressed ......   other ......

Pain Management Strategies:

☐ deep breathing ☐ meditation
☐ visualization ☐ one object focus
☐ calming scents ☐ PMR
☐ rest ☐ music

Something that made me smile:
....
....
Something I am proud of: ....
....
Something I am grateful for: ....
....
....
Something I am looking forward to: ....
....
....
Lowest pain level today: 1 2 3 4 5
Highest pain level today: 1 2 3 4 5

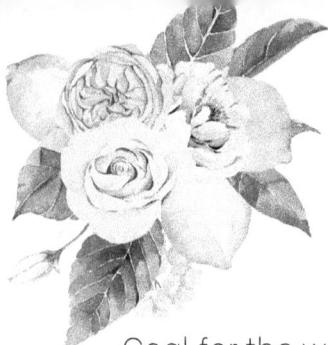

Week Eight

Goal for the week: ....
....

Days/Times I will leave the house or change settings: ....
....

When I will interact with friends or family: ....
....

Hobby I will work on: ....

Something new I'll try: ....

Medical tasks to do : ....
....
....

Monday........................

Sleep rating: 1 2 3 4 5

Mindset goal: ....
....

Eating goal: ....
....

Personal hygiene: bathe ......   teeth ......
style hair ......   get dressed ......   other ......

Pain Management Strategies:

☐ deep breathing ☐ meditation
☐ visualization ☐ one object focus
☐ calming scents ☐ PMR
☐ rest ☐ music

Something that made me smile:
....
....
Something I am proud of: ....
....
Something I am grateful for: ....
....
Something I am looking forward to: ....
....
....
Lowest pain level today: 1 2 3 4 5
Highest pain level today: 1 2 3 4 5

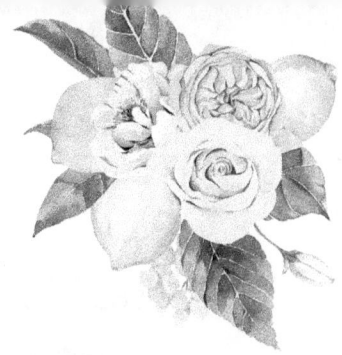

Week Eight

Tuesday.........................

Sleep rating: 1 2 3 4 5

Mindset goal: ....
....

Eating goal: ....
....

Personal hygiene: bathe ......   teeth ......
style hair ......   get dressed ......   other ......

Pain Management Strategies:

☐ deep breathing   ☐ meditation
☐ visualization   ☐ one object focus
☐ calming scents   ☐ PMR
☐ rest   ☐ music

Something that made me smile:
....
....
Something I am proud of: ....
....
Something I am grateful for: ....
....
Something I am looking forward to: ....
....
....

Lowest pain level today: 1 2 3 4 5
Highest pain level today: 1 2 3 4 5

Wednesday.........................

Sleep rating: 1 2 3 4 5

Mindset goal: ....
....

Eating goal: ....
....

Personal hygiene: bathe ......   teeth ......
style hair ......   get dressed ......   other ......

Pain Management Strategies:

☐ deep breathing   ☐ meditation
☐ visualization   ☐ one object focus
☐ calming scents   ☐ PMR
☐ rest   ☐ music

Something that made me smile:
....
....
Something I am proud of: ....
....
Something I am grateful for: ....
....
....
Something I am looking forward to: ....
....
....

Lowest pain level today: 1 2 3 4 5
Highest pain level today: 1 2 3 4 5

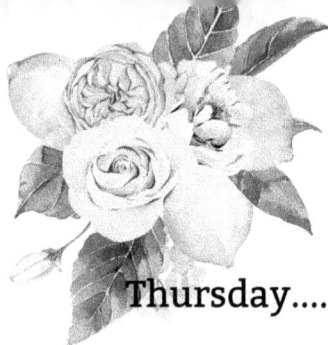

Week Eight

Thursday.....................

Sleep rating: 1 2 3 4 5

Mindset goal: ....
....

Eating goal: ....
....

Personal hygiene: bathe ......   teeth ......
style hair ......   get dressed ......   other ......

Pain Management Strategies:

☐ deep breathing ☐ meditation
☐ visualization   ☐ one object focus
☐ calming scents ☐ PMR
☐ rest   ☐ music

Something that made me smile:
....
....

Something I am proud of: ....
....

Something I am grateful for: ....
....

Something I am looking forward to: ....
....
....

Lowest pain level today: 1 2 3 4 5
Highest pain level today: 1 2 3 4 5

Friday..........................

Sleep rating: 1 2 3 4 5

Mindset goal: ....
....

Eating goal: ....
....

Personal hygiene: bathe ......   teeth ......
style hair ......   get dressed ......   other ......

Pain Management Strategies:

☐ deep breathing ☐ meditation
☐ visualization   ☐ one object focus
☐ calming scents ☐ PMR
☐ rest   ☐ music

Something that made me smile:
....
....

Something I am proud of: ....
....

Something I am grateful for: ....
....

Something I am looking forward to: ....
....
....

Lowest pain level today: 1 2 3 4 5
Highest pain level today: 1 2 3 4 5

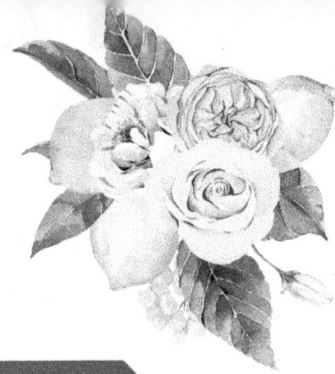

Saturday.....................

Sleep rating: 1 2 3 4 5

Mindset goal: ....
....

Eating goal: ....
....

Personal hygiene: bathe ...... teeth ......
style hair ...... get dressed ...... other ......

Pain Management Strategies:

☐ deep breathing ☐ meditation
☐ visualization ☐ one object focus
☐ calming scents ☐ PMR
☐ rest ☐ music

Something that made me smile:
....
....
Something I am proud of: ....
....
Something I am grateful for: ....
....
Something I am looking forward to: ....
....
....
Lowest pain level today: 1 2 3 4 5
Highest pain level today: 1 2 3 4 5

Sunday........................

Sleep rating: 1 2 3 4 5

Mindset goal: ....
....

Eating goal: ....
....

Personal hygiene: bathe ...... teeth ......
style hair ...... get dressed ...... other ......

Pain Management Strategies:

☐ deep breathing ☐ meditation
☐ visualization ☐ one object focus
☐ calming scents ☐ PMR
☐ rest ☐ music

Something that made me smile:
....
....
Something I am proud of: ....
....
Something I am grateful for: ....
....
....
Something I am looking forward to: ....
....
....
Lowest pain level today: 1 2 3 4 5
Highest pain level today: 1 2 3 4 5

Monthly Reflection

Think about how your mental health was this month. Did you use the strategies? When were you your best? Your worst?

....

....

....

....

....

....

....

....

....

....

....

....

....

....

....

....

....

....

....

Happy Distraction

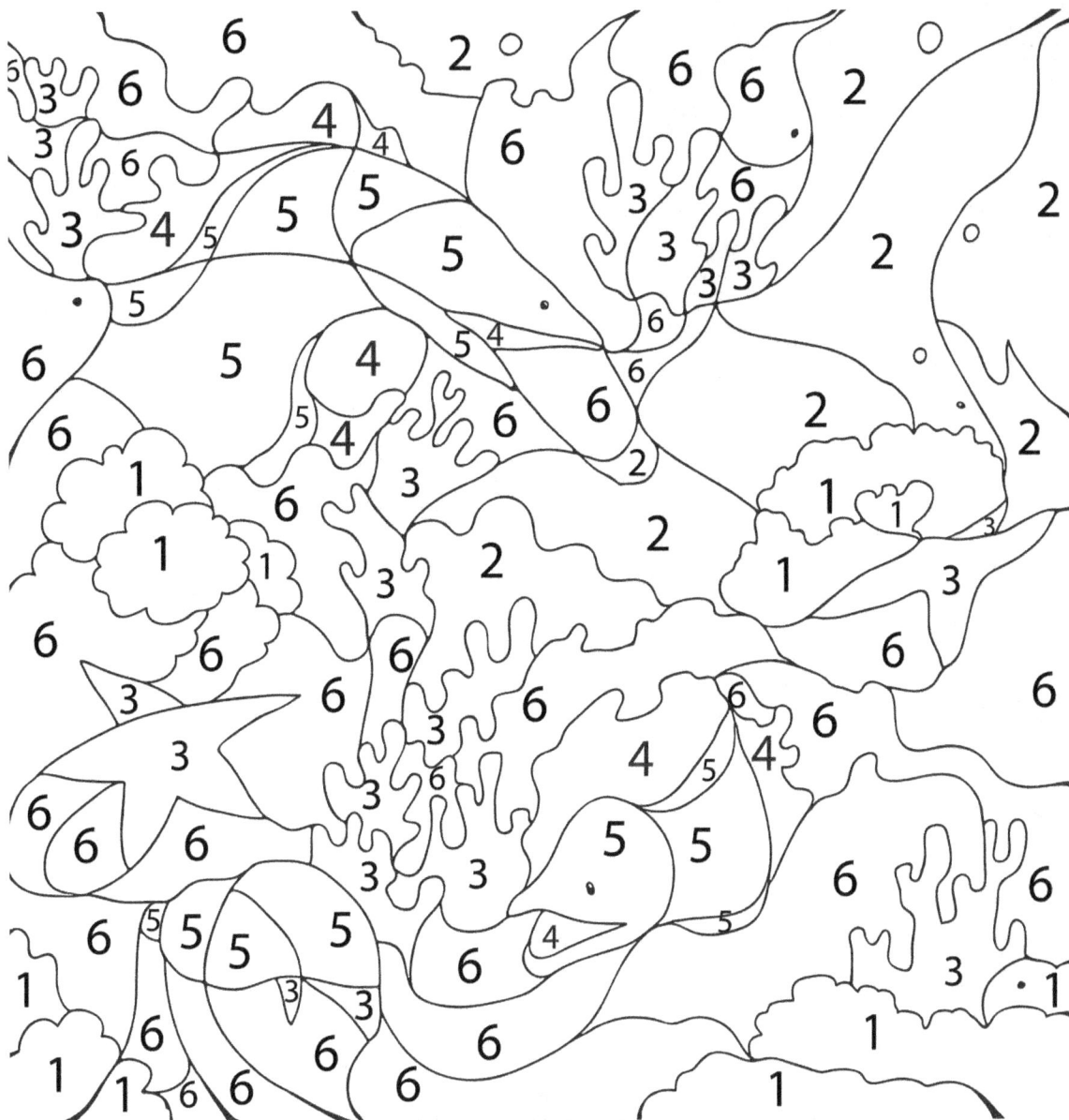

1 = light brown   2 = blue   3 = red   4 = black   5 = dark yellow   6 = green

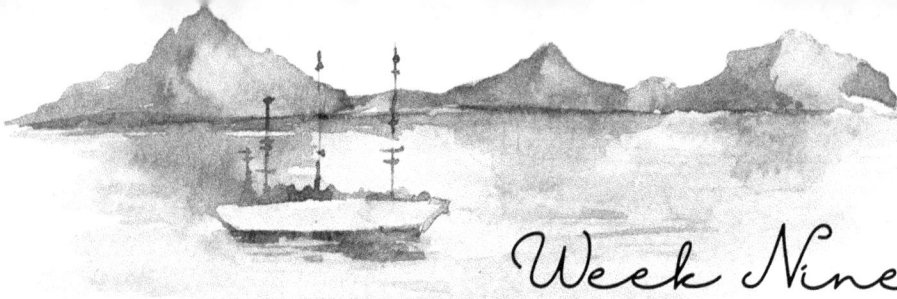

Week Nine

Goal for the week: ....
....

Days/Times I will leave the house or change settings: ....
....

When I will interact with friends or family: ....
....

Hobby I will work on: ....

Something new I'll try: ....

Medical tasks to do : ....
....
....

Monday........................

Sleep rating: 1 2 3 4 5

Mindset goal: ....
....

Eating goal: ....
....

Personal hygiene: bathe ...... teeth ......
style hair ...... get dressed ...... other ......

Pain Management Strategies:

☐ deep breathing ☐ meditation
☐ visualization ☐ one object focus
☐ calming scents ☐ PMR
☐ rest ☐ music

Something that made me smile:
....
....

Something I am proud of: ....
....

Something I am grateful for: ....
....

Something I am looking forward to: ....
....
....

Lowest pain level today: 1 2 3 4 5
Highest pain level today: 1 2 3 4 5

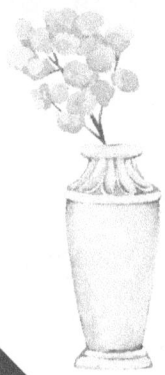

Tuesday..........................

Sleep rating: 1 2 3 4 5

Mindset goal: ....
....

Eating goal: ....
....

Personal hygiene: bathe ......   teeth ......
style hair ......   get dressed ......   other ......

Pain Management Strategies:

☐ deep breathing ☐ meditation
☐ visualization ☐ one object focus
☐ calming scents ☐ PMR
☐ rest ☐ music

Something that made me smile:
....
....
Something I am proud of: ....
....
Something I am grateful for: ....
....
Something I am looking forward to: ....
....
....
Lowest pain level today: 1 2 3 4 5
Highest pain level today: 1 2 3 4 5

Wednesday..........................

Sleep rating: 1 2 3 4 5

Mindset goal: ....
....

Eating goal: ....
....

Personal hygiene: bathe ......   teeth ......
style hair ......   get dressed ......   other ......

Pain Management Strategies:

☐ deep breathing ☐ meditation
☐ visualization ☐ one object focus
☐ calming scents ☐ PMR
☐ rest ☐ music

Something that made me smile:
....
....
Something I am proud of: ....
....
Something I am grateful for: ....
....
Something I am looking forward to: ....
....
....
Lowest pain level today: 1 2 3 4 5
Highest pain level today: 1 2 3 4 5

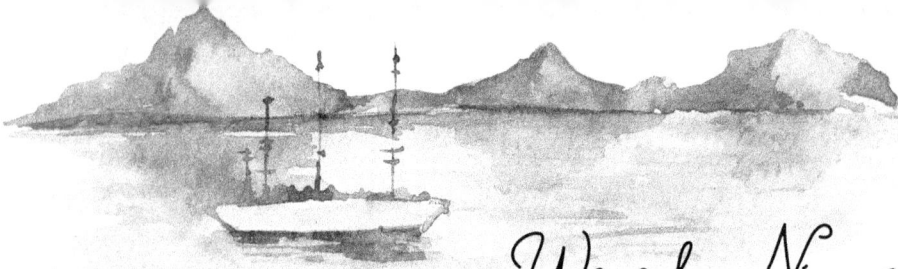

Thursday........................

Sleep rating: 1 2 3 4 5

Mindset goal: ....
....

Eating goal: ....
....

Personal hygiene: bathe ......   teeth ......
style hair ......   get dressed ......   other ......

Pain Management Strategies:

☐ deep breathing   ☐ meditation
☐ visualization   ☐ one object focus
☐ calming scents   ☐ PMR
☐ rest   ☐ music

Something that made me smile:
....
....

Something I am proud of: ....
....

Something I am grateful for: ....
....

Something I am looking forward to: ....
....
....

Lowest pain level today: 1 2 3 4 5
Highest pain level today: 1 2 3 4 5

Friday...........................

Sleep rating: 1 2 3 4 5

Mindset goal: ....
....

Eating goal: ....
....

Personal hygiene: bathe ......   teeth ......
style hair ......   get dressed ......   other ......

Pain Management Strategies:

☐ deep breathing   ☐ meditation
☐ visualization   ☐ one object focus
☐ calming scents   ☐ PMR
☐ rest   ☐ music

Something that made me smile:
....
....

Something I am proud of: ....
....

Something I am grateful for: ....
....

Something I am looking forward to: ....
....
....

Lowest pain level today: 1 2 3 4 5
Highest pain level today: 1 2 3 4 5

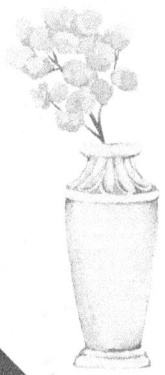

Week Nine

Saturday........................

Sleep rating: 1 2 3 4 5

Mindset goal: ....
....

Eating goal: ....
....

Personal hygiene: bathe ......   teeth ......
style hair ......   get dressed ......   other ......

Pain Management Strategies:

☐ deep breathing ☐ meditation
☐ visualization ☐ one object focus
☐ calming scents ☐ PMR
☐ rest ☐ music

Something that made me smile:
....
....
Something I am proud of: ....
....
Something I am grateful for: ....
....
Something I am looking forward to: ....
....
....
Lowest pain level today: 1 2 3 4 5
Highest pain level today: 1 2 3 4 5

Sunday..........................

Sleep rating: 1 2 3 4 5

Mindset goal: ....
....

Eating goal: ....
....

Personal hygiene: bathe ......   teeth ......
style hair ......   get dressed ......   other ......

Pain Management Strategies:

☐ deep breathing ☐ meditation
☐ visualization ☐ one object focus
☐ calming scents ☐ PMR
☐ rest ☐ music

Something that made me smile:
....
....
Something I am proud of: ....
....
Something I am grateful for: ....
....
....
Something I am looking forward to: ....
....
....
Lowest pain level today: 1 2 3 4 5
Highest pain level today: 1 2 3 4 5

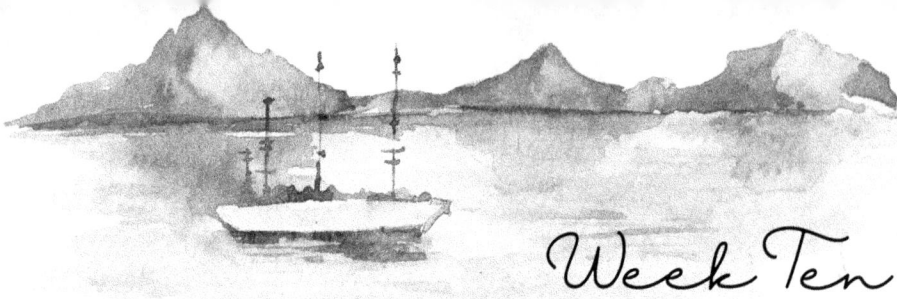

Week Ten

Goal for the week: ....
....

Days/Times I will leave the house or change settings: ....
....

When I will interact with friends or family: ....
....

Hobby I will work on: ....

Something new I'll try: ....

Medical tasks to do : ....
....
....

Monday.........................

Sleep rating: 1 2 3 4 5

Mindset goal: ....
....

Eating goal: ....
....

Personal hygiene: bathe ......   teeth ......
style hair ......   get dressed ......   other ......

Pain Management Strategies:

- [ ] deep breathing
- [ ] visualization
- [ ] calming scents
- [ ] rest
- [ ] meditation
- [ ] one object focus
- [ ] PMR
- [ ] music

Something that made me smile:
....
....
Something I am proud of: ....
....
Something I am grateful for: ....
....
Something I am looking forward to: ....
....
....

Lowest pain level today: 1 2 3 4 5
Highest pain level today: 1 2 3 4 5

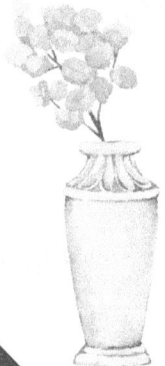

Week Ten

Tuesday......................

Sleep rating: 1 2 3 4 5

Mindset goal: ....
....

Eating goal: ....
....

Personal hygiene: bathe ......   teeth ......
style hair ......   get dressed ......   other ......

Pain Management Strategies:

☐ deep breathing ☐ meditation
☐ visualization   ☐ one object focus
☐ calming scents ☐ PMR
☐ rest   ☐ music

Something that made me smile:
....
....
Something I am proud of: ....
....
Something I am grateful for: ....
....
Something I am looking forward to: ....
....
....

Lowest pain level today: 1 2 3 4 5
Highest pain level today: 1 2 3 4 5

Wednesday........................

Sleep rating: 1 2 3 4 5

Mindset goal: ....
....

Eating goal: ....
....

Personal hygiene: bathe ......   teeth ......
style hair ......   get dressed ......   other ......

Pain Management Strategies:

☐ deep breathing ☐ meditation
☐ visualization   ☐ one object focus
☐ calming scents ☐ PMR
☐ rest   ☐ music

Something that made me smile:
....
....
Something I am proud of: ....
....
Something I am grateful for: ....
....
Something I am looking forward to: ....
....
....

Lowest pain level today: 1 2 3 4 5
Highest pain level today: 1 2 3 4 5

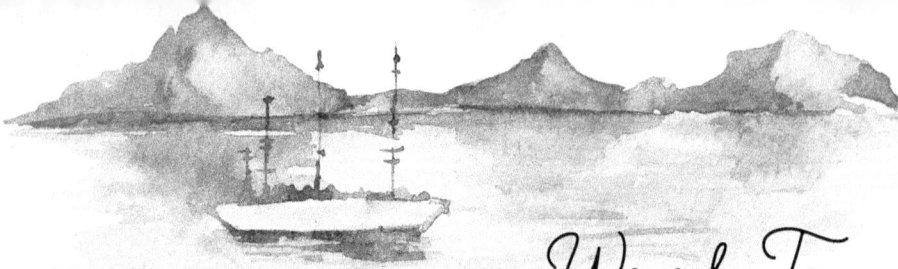

Thursday.....................

Sleep rating: 1 2 3 4 5

Mindset goal: ....
....

Eating goal: ....
....

Personal hygiene: bathe ...... teeth ......
style hair ...... get dressed ...... other ......

Pain Management Strategies:

- ☐ deep breathing ☐ meditation
- ☐ visualization ☐ one object focus
- ☐ calming scents ☐ PMR
- ☐ rest ☐ music

Something that made me smile:
....
....

Something I am proud of: ....
....

Something I am grateful for: ....
....

Something I am looking forward to: ....
....
....

Lowest pain level today: 1 2 3 4 5
Highest pain level today: 1 2 3 4 5

Friday.........................

Sleep rating: 1 2 3 4 5

Mindset goal: ....
....

Eating goal: ....
....

Personal hygiene: bathe ...... teeth ......
style hair ...... get dressed ...... other ......

Pain Management Strategies:

- ☐ deep breathing ☐ meditation
- ☐ visualization ☐ one object focus
- ☐ calming scents ☐ PMR
- ☐ rest ☐ music

Something that made me smile:
....
....

Something I am proud of: ....
....

Something I am grateful for: ....
....

Something I am looking forward to: ....
....
....

Lowest pain level today: 1 2 3 4 5
Highest pain level today: 1 2 3 4 5

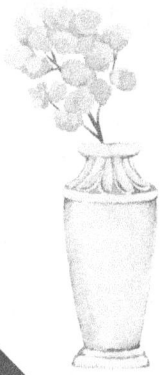

Week Ten

Saturday......................

Sleep rating: 1 2 3 4 5

Mindset goal: ....
....

Eating goal: ....
....

Personal hygiene: bathe ......   teeth ......
style hair ......   get dressed ......   other ......

Pain Management Strategies:

☐ deep breathing ☐ meditation
☐ visualization ☐ one object focus
☐ calming scents ☐ PMR
☐ rest ☐ music

Something that made me smile:
....
....
Something I am proud of: ....
....
Something I am grateful for: ....
....
Something I am looking forward to: ....
....
....
Lowest pain level today: 1 2 3 4 5
Highest pain level today: 1 2 3 4 5

Sunday.........................

Sleep rating: 1 2 3 4 5

Mindset goal: ....
....

Eating goal: ....
....

Personal hygiene: bathe ......   teeth ......
style hair ......   get dressed ......   other ......

Pain Management Strategies:

☐ deep breathing ☐ meditation
☐ visualization ☐ one object focus
☐ calming scents ☐ PMR
☐ rest ☐ music

Something that made me smile:
....
....
Something I am proud of: ....
....
Something I am grateful for: ....
....
....
Something I am looking forward to: ....
....
....
Lowest pain level today: 1 2 3 4 5
Highest pain level today: 1 2 3 4 5

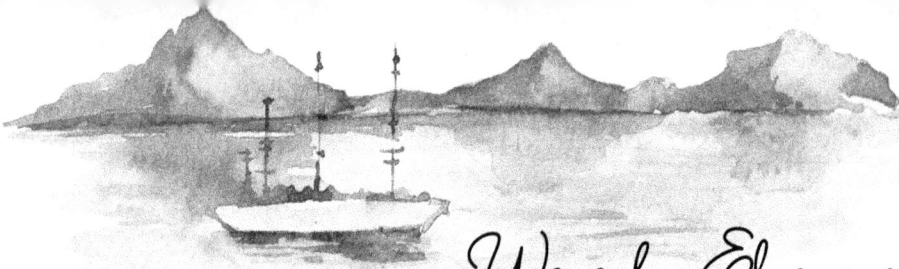

Week Eleven

Goal for the week: ....
....

Days/Times I will leave the house or change settings: ....
....

When I will interact with friends or family: ....
....

Hobby I will work on: ....

Something new I'll try: ....

Medical tasks to do : ....
....
....

Monday.........................

Sleep rating: 1 2 3 4 5

Mindset goal: ....
....

Eating goal: ....
....

Personal hygiene: bathe ...... teeth ......
style hair ......   get dressed ......   other ......

Pain Management Strategies:

☐ deep breathing ☐ meditation
☐ visualization   ☐ one object focus
☐ calming scents ☐ PMR
☐ rest   ☐ music

Something that made me smile:
....
....
Something I am proud of: ....
....
Something I am grateful for: ....
....
....
Something I am looking forward to: ....
....
....
Lowest pain level today: 1 2 3 4 5
Highest pain level today: 1 2 3 4 5

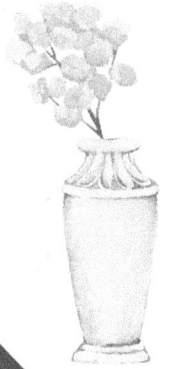

Week Eleven

Tuesday..........................

Sleep rating: 1 2 3 4 5

Mindset goal: ....
....

Eating goal: ....
....

Personal hygiene: bathe ......   teeth ......
style hair ......   get dressed ......   other ......

Pain Management Strategies:

☐ deep breathing ☐ meditation
☐ visualization   ☐ one object focus
☐ calming scents ☐ PMR
☐ rest   ☐ music

Something that made me smile:
....
....
Something I am proud of: ....
....
Something I am grateful for: ....
....
Something I am looking forward to: ....
....
....
Lowest pain level today: 1 2 3 4 5
Highest pain level today: 1 2 3 4 5

Wednesday..........................

Sleep rating: 1 2 3 4 5

Mindset goal: ....
....

Eating goal: ....
....

Personal hygiene: bathe ......   teeth ......
style hair ......   get dressed ......   other ......

Pain Management Strategies:

☐ deep breathing ☐ meditation
☐ visualization   ☐ one object focus
☐ calming scents ☐ PMR
☐ rest   ☐ music

Something that made me smile:
....
....
Something I am proud of: ....
....
Something I am grateful for: ....
....
....
Something I am looking forward to: ....
....
....
Lowest pain level today: 1 2 3 4 5
Highest pain level today: 1 2 3 4 5

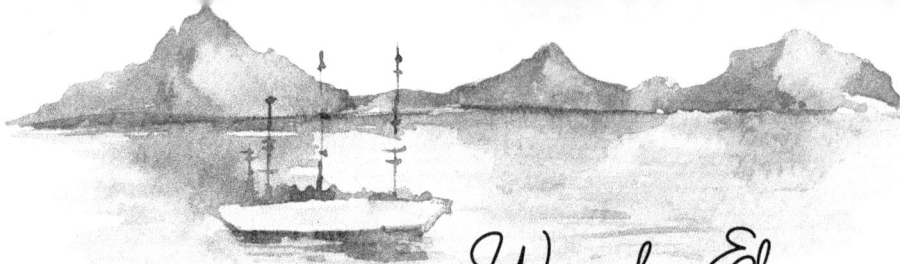

Sleep rating: 1 2 3 4 5

Mindset goal: ....
....

Eating goal: ....
....

Personal hygiene: bathe ...... teeth ......
style hair ...... get dressed ...... other ......

Pain Management Strategies:

☐ deep breathing ☐ meditation
☐ visualization ☐ one object focus
☐ calming scents ☐ PMR
☐ rest ☐ music

Something that made me smile:
....
....
Something I am proud of: ....
....
Something I am grateful for: ....
....
Something I am looking forward to: ....
....
....

Lowest pain level today: 1 2 3 4 5
Highest pain level today: 1 2 3 4 5

Friday.........................

Sleep rating: 1 2 3 4 5

Mindset goal: ....
....

Eating goal: ....
....

Personal hygiene: bathe ...... teeth ......
style hair ...... get dressed ...... other ......

Pain Management Strategies:

☐ deep breathing ☐ meditation
☐ visualization ☐ one object focus
☐ calming scents ☐ PMR
☐ rest ☐ music

Something that made me smile:
....
....
Something I am proud of: ....
....
Something I am grateful for: ....
....
Something I am looking forward to: ....
....
....

Lowest pain level today: 1 2 3 4 5
Highest pain level today: 1 2 3 4 5

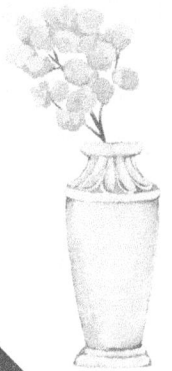

Week Eleven

Saturday........................

Sleep rating: 1 2 3 4 5

Mindset goal: ....

....

Eating goal: ....

....

Personal hygiene: bathe ......   teeth ......
style hair ......   get dressed ......   other ......

Pain Management Strategies:

☐ deep breathing   ☐ meditation
☐ visualization   ☐ one object focus
☐ calming scents   ☐ PMR
☐ rest   ☐ music

Something that made me smile:
....
....
Something I am proud of: ....
....
....
Something I am grateful for: ....
....
....
Something I am looking forward to: ....
....
....
Lowest pain level today: 1 2 3 4 5
Highest pain level today: 1 2 3 4 5

Sunday........................

Sleep rating: 1 2 3 4 5

Mindset goal: ....

....

Eating goal: ....

....

Personal hygiene: bathe ......   teeth ......
style hair ......   get dressed ......   other ......

Pain Management Strategies:

☐ deep breathing   ☐ meditation
☐ visualization   ☐ one object focus
☐ calming scents   ☐ PMR
☐ rest   ☐ music

Something that made me smile:
....
....
Something I am proud of: ....
....
....
Something I am grateful for: ....
....
....
Something I am looking forward to: ....
....
....
Lowest pain level today: 1 2 3 4 5
Highest pain level today: 1 2 3 4 5

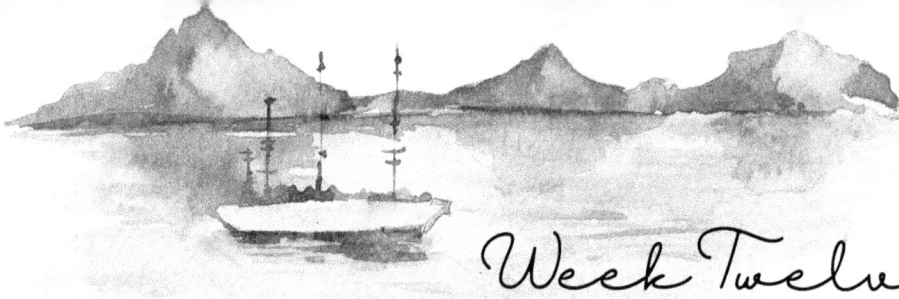

Week Twelve

Goal for the week: ....
....

Days/Times I will leave the house or change settings: ....
....

When I will interact with friends or family: ....
....

Hobby I will work on: ....

Something new I'll try: ....

Medical tasks to do : ....
....
....

Monday........................

Sleep rating: 1 2 3 4 5

Mindset goal: ....
....

Eating goal: ....
....

Personal hygiene: bathe ......   teeth ......
style hair ......   get dressed ......   other ......

Pain Management Strategies:

- [ ] deep breathing [ ] meditation
- [ ] visualization [ ] one object focus
- [ ] calming scents [ ] PMR
- [ ] rest [ ] music

Something that made me smile:
....
....
Something I am proud of: ....
....
Something I am grateful for: ....
....
....
Something I am looking forward to: ....
....
....

Lowest pain level today: 1 2 3 4 5
Highest pain level today: 1 2 3 4 5

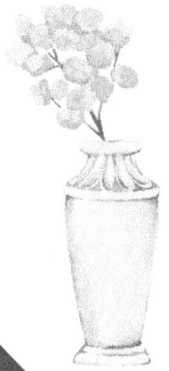

Week Twelve

Tuesday.........................

Sleep rating: 1 2 3 4 5

Mindset goal: ....
....

Eating goal: ....
....

Personal hygiene: bathe ...... teeth ......
style hair ...... get dressed ...... other ......

Pain Management Strategies:

- [ ] deep breathing
- [ ] visualization
- [ ] calming scents
- [ ] rest
- [ ] meditation
- [ ] one object focus
- [ ] PMR
- [ ] music

Something that made me smile:
....
....

Something I am proud of: ....
....

Something I am grateful for: ....
....

Something I am looking forward to: ....
....

Lowest pain level today: 1 2 3 4 5
Highest pain level today: 1 2 3 4 5

Wednesday.........................

Sleep rating: 1 2 3 4 5

Mindset goal: ....
....

Eating goal: ....
....

Personal hygiene: bathe ...... teeth ......
style hair ...... get dressed ...... other ......

Pain Management Strategies:

- [ ] deep breathing
- [ ] visualization
- [ ] calming scents
- [ ] rest
- [ ] meditation
- [ ] one object focus
- [ ] PMR
- [ ] music

Something that made me smile:
....
....

Something I am proud of: ....
....

Something I am grateful for: ....
....

Something I am looking forward to: ....
....

Lowest pain level today: 1 2 3 4 5
Highest pain level today: 1 2 3 4 5

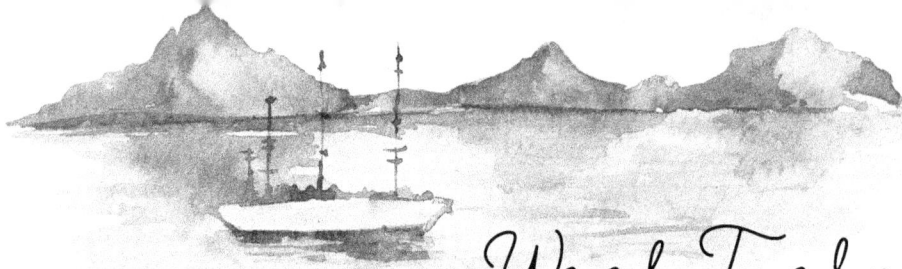

Thursday.....................

Sleep rating: 1 2 3 4 5

Mindset goal: ....
....

Eating goal: ....
....

Personal hygiene: bathe ......   teeth ......
style hair ......   get dressed ......   other ......

Pain Management Strategies:

- ☐ deep breathing ☐ meditation
- ☐ visualization ☐ one object focus
- ☐ calming scents ☐ PMR
- ☐ rest ☐ music

Something that made me smile:
....
....

Something I am proud of: ....

Something I am grateful for: ....

Something I am looking forward to: ....

Lowest pain level today: 1 2 3 4 5
Highest pain level today: 1 2 3 4 5

Friday.........................

Sleep rating: 1 2 3 4 5

Mindset goal: ....
....

Eating goal: ....
....

Personal hygiene: bathe ......   teeth ......
style hair ......   get dressed ......   other ......

Pain Management Strategies:

- ☐ deep breathing ☐ meditation
- ☐ visualization ☐ one object focus
- ☐ calming scents ☐ PMR
- ☐ rest ☐ music

Something that made me smile:
....
....

Something I am proud of: ....

Something I am grateful for: ....

Something I am looking forward to: ....

Lowest pain level today: 1 2 3 4 5
Highest pain level today: 1 2 3 4 5

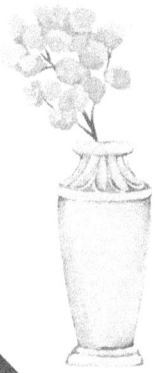

Week Twelve

Saturday........................

Sleep rating: 1 2 3 4 5

Mindset goal: ....
....

Eating goal: ....
....

Personal hygiene: bathe ...... teeth ......
style hair ...... get dressed ...... other ......

Pain Management Strategies:

☐ deep breathing ☐ meditation
☐ visualization ☐ one object focus
☐ calming scents ☐ PMR
☐ rest ☐ music

Something that made me smile:
....
....

Something I am proud of: ....
....

Something I am grateful for: ....
....

Something I am looking forward to: ....
....
....

Lowest pain level today: 1 2 3 4 5
Highest pain level today: 1 2 3 4 5

Sunday........................

Sleep rating: 1 2 3 4 5

Mindset goal: ....
....

Eating goal: ....
....

Personal hygiene: bathe ...... teeth ......
style hair ...... get dressed ...... other ......

Pain Management Strategies:

☐ deep breathing ☐ meditation
☐ visualization ☐ one object focus
☐ calming scents ☐ PMR
☐ rest ☐ music

Something that made me smile:
....
....

Something I am proud of: ....
....

Something I am grateful for: ....
....

Something I am looking forward to: ....
....
....

Lowest pain level today: 1 2 3 4 5
Highest pain level today: 1 2 3 4 5

Monthly Reflection

Think about how your mental health was this month. Did you use the strategies?
When were you your best? Your worst?

....

....

....

....

....

....

....

....

....

....

....

....

....

....

....

Happy Distraction

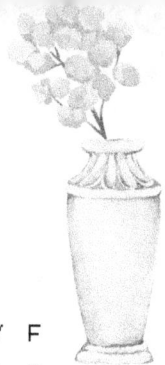

```
X X M J A H Y V P X V B N T E T S A H K N Z M I T M B S V F
R I X R C G N O T O U V S O T X K C Z T O K U M Z U C Y G C
Y O M N I K H H X T P R F X A N I F T W D V G D I S V Y D P
L F U F C H K T P U Y E E L Q T C B H V L M U M K V B Z H
G R F Q A N O E M B J O L Q O G T L I C O R I C E E H U J V
C U A A E U R I R B Q D X L C G L Z A K M K P P I T J J U V
O P M R T S V A I Q J X M B O V E M F X Y Y E G N E G M O O
U E D M C V T T K J B T V H H L S L J S F Z G I O E G H O
B S I O I S T U L F A P U W C U I G Z Z G X B O Y R S W S K
Z D T S U E D Y H I B Z L Z B A F K D L V P Y E O S F T C F
R C V F T F S C V M E N O R K O M X D E B J M X V R Q N L Q
H G B O Y O G L O L P C Q K K Y U O M N K O G M S J D F P E
O N H F A X O L L P S P O N Y R H K H K D Z W I Q N K A S Y
P T R A B N M T S V U T M L J V Z R V M U Y S R E K C I N S
X S Y Q W P O M H S R E G N I F R E T T U B Z L P K B T I I
O X F F W S C O L E Q V X B F T B G T X G A Q C Q Z U W T S
I S D F C C O M K S G H D A A N M E R F K M Z N B D C A J L
B H K R V E T O K S W G K H O V K X O T J S E A U G G E R Y
O A I Y B H S W L I D A Z V R A T Q W V Y U U M H U F B D O
Y D T T A O Q Q I K C A R A M E L I I Z C P I U I F I E H G
X L K O U K R B O X M Q S H Y X G G P K F H U Q Z O I Y X W
F B A R V O D U L I V H H H Y L K G D E T K Z S I A Q E P B
S Z T I R L E L Q Q G B N Q Q B S Y Y N S K D W Z M U K O
R N R D Y B V M D S E T Q R V E D P H U Y J D Q W X K Y C B
B N C G U Q Z P D A E T C O S I E J L M J D H C C E G T N S
Q X Z T H E R S H E Y R I E M F C I F L X M S P V Y P V N E
T R M N U D J Q D D G Y E S I M O U X Z U W A J Y E S L J P
T E Q Y K J N F Q Q K R F D R W E O F M N G G P K T H M V Z
P T B Q C U D V P A V O P Q M J M P S Z M B P D N D A O Q G
P G O P M V Z Y E B Z L F U G B Q T H C T A P C L A L Q T S
```

Candy

butterfinger butterscotch caramel chocolate crunch gum gummies
hershey kisses kitkat licorice lollypop musketeers nerds nestle
sour patch reeses skittles snickers starburst taffy tootsie twix

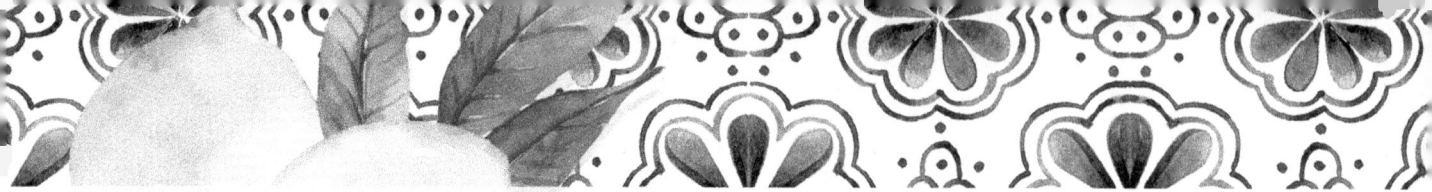

Week Thirteen

Goal for the week: ....
....

Days/Times I will leave the house or change settings: ....
....

When I will interact with friends or family: ....
....

Hobby I will work on: ....

Something new I'll try: ....

Medical tasks to do : ....
....
....

Monday...........................

Sleep rating: 1   2   3   4   5

Mindset goal: ....
....

Eating goal: ....
....

Personal hygiene: bathe ......   teeth ......
style hair ......   get dressed ......   other ......

Pain Management Strategies:

- [ ] deep breathing
- [ ] visualization
- [ ] calming scents
- [ ] rest
- [ ] meditation
- [ ] one object focus
- [ ] PMR
- [ ] music

Something that made me smile:
....
....

Something I am proud of: ....
....

Something I am grateful for: ....
....
....

Something I am looking forward to: ....
....
....

Lowest pain level today: 1 2 3 4 5
Highest pain level today: 1 2 3 4 5

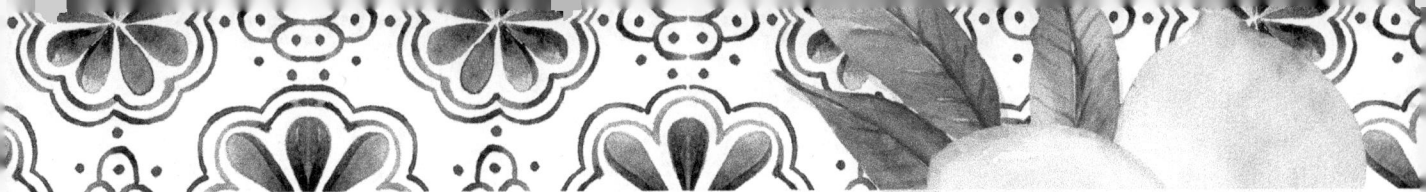

Week Thirteen

Tuesday..........................

Sleep rating: 1 2 3 4 5

Mindset goal: ....
....

Eating goal: ....
....

Personal hygiene: bathe ...... teeth ......
style hair ...... get dressed ...... other ......

Pain Management Strategies:

☐ deep breathing ☐ meditation
☐ visualization ☐ one object focus
☐ calming scents ☐ PMR
☐ rest ☐ music

Something that made me smile:
....
....
Something I am proud of: ....
....
Something I am grateful for: ....
....
Something I am looking forward to: ....
....
....

Lowest pain level today: 1 2 3 4 5
Highest pain level today: 1 2 3 4 5

Wednesday...........................

Sleep rating: 1 2 3 4 5

Mindset goal: ....
....

Eating goal: ....
....

Personal hygiene: bathe ...... teeth ......
style hair ...... get dressed ...... other ......

Pain Management Strategies:

☐ deep breathing ☐ meditation
☐ visualization ☐ one object focus
☐ calming scents ☐ PMR
☐ rest ☐ music

Something that made me smile:
....
....
Something I am proud of: ....
....
Something I am grateful for: ....
....
Something I am looking forward to: ....
....
....

Lowest pain level today: 1 2 3 4 5
Highest pain level today: 1 2 3 4 5

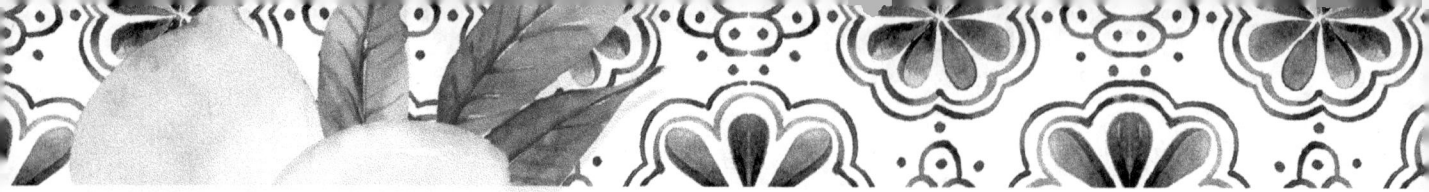

Week Thirteen

Thursday.....................

Sleep rating: 1 2 3 4 5

Mindset goal: ....
....

Eating goal: ....
....

Personal hygiene: bathe ......   teeth ......
style hair ......   get dressed ......   other ......

Pain Management Strategies:

- [ ] deep breathing [ ] meditation
- [ ] visualization [ ] one object focus
- [ ] calming scents [ ] PMR
- [ ] rest [ ] music

Something that made me smile:
....
....

Something I am proud of: ....
....

Something I am grateful for: ....
....

Something I am looking forward to: ....
....
....

Lowest pain level today: 1 2 3 4 5
Highest pain level today: 1 2 3 4 5

Friday.........................

Sleep rating: 1 2 3 4 5

Mindset goal: ....
....

Eating goal: ....
....

Personal hygiene: bathe ......   teeth ......
style hair ......   get dressed ......   other ......

Pain Management Strategies:

- [ ] deep breathing [ ] meditation
- [ ] visualization [ ] one object focus
- [ ] calming scents [ ] PMR
- [ ] rest [ ] music

Something that made me smile:
....
....

Something I am proud of: ....
....

Something I am grateful for: ....
....

Something I am looking forward to: ....
....
....

Lowest pain level today: 1 2 3 4 5
Highest pain level today: 1 2 3 4 5

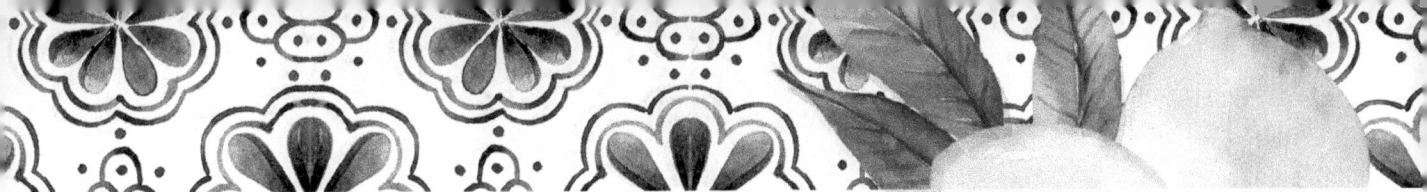

Week Thirteen

Saturday......................

Sleep rating: 1 2 3 4 5

Mindset goal: ....
....

Eating goal: ....
....

Personal hygiene: bathe ...... teeth ......
style hair ...... get dressed ...... other ......

Pain Management Strategies:

☐ deep breathing ☐ meditation
☐ visualization ☐ one object focus
☐ calming scents ☐ PMR
☐ rest ☐ music

Something that made me smile:
....
....
Something I am proud of: ....
....
Something I am grateful for: ....
....
Something I am looking forward to: ....
....
....

Lowest pain level today: 1 2 3 4 5
Highest pain level today: 1 2 3 4 5

Sunday........................

Sleep rating: 1 2 3 4 5

Mindset goal: ....
....

Eating goal: ....
....

Personal hygiene: bathe ...... teeth ......
style hair ...... get dressed ...... other ......

Pain Management Strategies:

☐ deep breathing ☐ meditation
☐ visualization ☐ one object focus
☐ calming scents ☐ PMR
☐ rest ☐ music

Something that made me smile:
....
....
Something I am proud of: ....
....
Something I am grateful for: ....
....
....
Something I am looking forward to: ....
....
....

Lowest pain level today: 1 2 3 4 5
Highest pain level today: 1 2 3 4 5

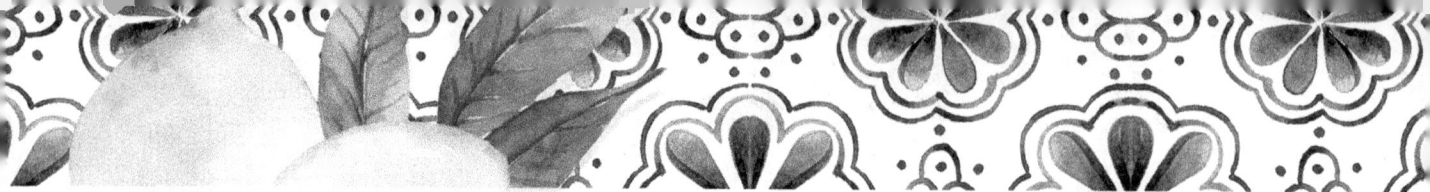

Week Fourteen

Goal for the week: ....
....

Days/Times I will leave the house or change settings: ....
....

When I will interact with friends or family: ....
....

Hobby I will work on: ....

Something new I'll try: ....

Medical tasks to do : ....
....
....

Monday........................

Sleep rating: 1 2 3 4 5

Mindset goal: ....
....

Eating goal: ....
....

Personal hygiene: bathe ......   teeth ......
style hair ......   get dressed ......   other ......

Pain Management Strategies:

☐ deep breathing ☐ meditation
☐ visualization ☐ one object focus
☐ calming scents ☐ PMR
☐ rest ☐ music

Something that made me smile:
....
....
Something I am proud of: ....
....
Something I am grateful for: ....
....
....
Something I am looking forward to: ....
....
....
Lowest pain level today: 1 2 3 4 5
Highest pain level today: 1 2 3 4 5

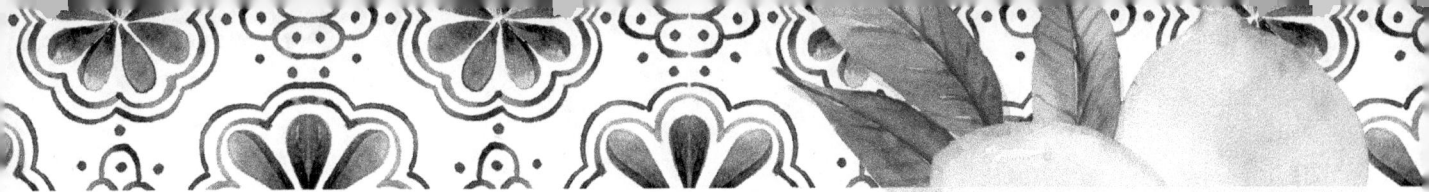

Tuesday...............................

Sleep rating: 1 2 3 4 5

Mindset goal: ....

....

Eating goal: ....

....

Personal hygiene: bathe ...... teeth ......
style hair ...... get dressed ...... other ......

Pain Management Strategies:

☐ deep breathing ☐ meditation
☐ visualization ☐ one object focus
☐ calming scents ☐ PMR
☐ rest ☐ music

Something that made me smile:

....

....

Something I am proud of: ....

....

Something I am grateful for: ....

....

Something I am looking forward to: ....

....

....

Lowest pain level today: 1 2 3 4 5
Highest pain level today: 1 2 3 4 5

Wednesday...........................

Sleep rating: 1 2 3 4 5

Mindset goal: ....

....

Eating goal: ....

....

Personal hygiene: bathe ...... teeth ......
style hair ...... get dressed ...... other ......

Pain Management Strategies:

☐ deep breathing ☐ meditation
☐ visualization ☐ one object focus
☐ calming scents ☐ PMR
☐ rest ☐ music

Something that made me smile:

....

....

Something I am proud of: ....

....

Something I am grateful for: ....

....

Something I am looking forward to: ....

....

....

Lowest pain level today: 1 2 3 4 5
Highest pain level today: 1 2 3 4 5

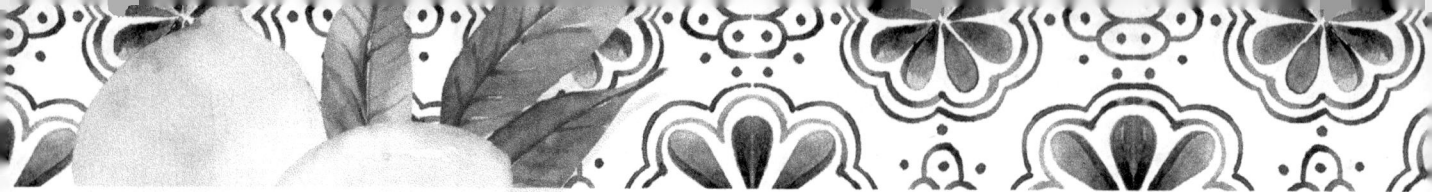

Thursday.....................

Sleep rating: 1 2 3 4 5

Mindset goal: ....
....

Eating goal: ....
....

Personal hygiene: bathe ...... teeth ......
style hair ...... get dressed ...... other ......

Pain Management Strategies:

☐ deep breathing ☐ meditation
☐ visualization ☐ one object focus
☐ calming scents ☐ PMR
☐ rest ☐ music

Something that made me smile:
....
....

Something I am proud of: ....
....

Something I am grateful for: ....
....

Something I am looking forward to: ....
....
....

Lowest pain level today: 1 2 3 4 5
Highest pain level today: 1 2 3 4 5

Friday..........................

Sleep rating: 1 2 3 4 5

Mindset goal: ....
....

Eating goal: ....
....

Personal hygiene: bathe ...... teeth ......
style hair ...... get dressed ...... other ......

Pain Management Strategies:

☐ deep breathing ☐ meditation
☐ visualization ☐ one object focus
☐ calming scents ☐ PMR
☐ rest ☐ music

Something that made me smile:
....
....

Something I am proud of: ....
....

Something I am grateful for: ....
....

Something I am looking forward to: ....
....
....

Lowest pain level today: 1 2 3 4 5
Highest pain level today: 1 2 3 4 5

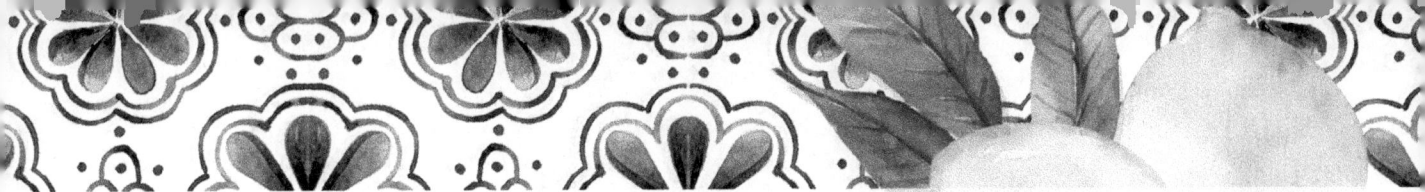

Saturday........................

Sleep rating: 1 2 3 4 5

Mindset goal: ....
....

Eating goal: ....
....

Personal hygiene: bathe ...... teeth ......
style hair ...... get dressed ...... other ......

Pain Management Strategies:

☐ deep breathing ☐ meditation
☐ visualization ☐ one object focus
☐ calming scents ☐ PMR
☐ rest ☐ music

Something that made me smile:
....
....
Something I am proud of: ....
....
Something I am grateful for: ....
....
Something I am looking forward to: ....
....
....
Lowest pain level today: 1 2 3 4 5
Highest pain level today: 1 2 3 4 5

Sunday..........................

Sleep rating: 1 2 3 4 5

Mindset goal: ....
....

Eating goal: ....
....

Personal hygiene: bathe ...... teeth ......
style hair ...... get dressed ...... other ......

Pain Management Strategies:

☐ deep breathing ☐ meditation
☐ visualization ☐ one object focus
☐ calming scents ☐ PMR
☐ rest ☐ music

Something that made me smile:
....
....
Something I am proud of: ....
....
Something I am grateful for: ....
....
....
Something I am looking forward to: ....
....
....
Lowest pain level today: 1 2 3 4 5
Highest pain level today: 1 2 3 4 5

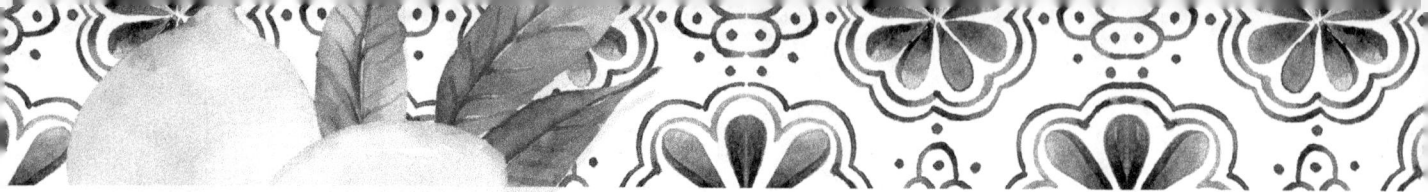

Week Fifteen

Goal for the week: ....
....

Days/Times I will leave the house or change settings: ....
....

When I will interact with friends or family: ....
....

Hobby I will work on: ....

Something new I'll try: ....

Medical tasks to do : ....
....
....

Monday..........................

Sleep rating: 1 2 3 4 5

Mindset goal: ....
....

Eating goal: ....
....

Personal hygiene: bathe ......   teeth ......
style hair ......   get dressed ......   other ......

Pain Management Strategies:

- [ ] deep breathing [ ] meditation
- [ ] visualization [ ] one object focus
- [ ] calming scents [ ] PMR
- [ ] rest [ ] music

Something that made me smile: ....
....
....
Something I am proud of: ....
....
Something I am grateful for: ....
....
Something I am looking forward to: ....
....
....

Lowest pain level today: 1 2 3 4 5
Highest pain level today: 1 2 3 4 5

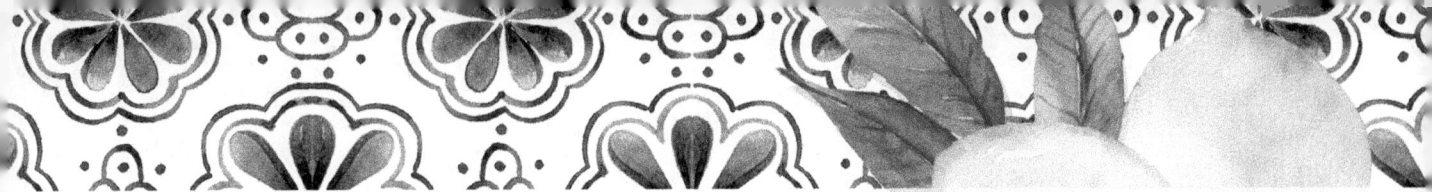

Week Fifteen

Tuesday.........................

Sleep rating: 1 2 3 4 5

Mindset goal: ....
....

Eating goal: ....
....

Personal hygiene: bathe ...... teeth ......
style hair ...... get dressed ...... other ......

Pain Management Strategies:

- [ ] deep breathing
- [ ] visualization
- [ ] calming scents
- [ ] rest
- [ ] meditation
- [ ] one object focus
- [ ] PMR
- [ ] music

Something that made me smile:
....
....
Something I am proud of: ....
....
Something I am grateful for: ....
....
....
Something I am looking forward to: ....
....
....

Lowest pain level today: 1 2 3 4 5
Highest pain level today: 1 2 3 4 5

Wednesday.........................

Sleep rating: 1 2 3 4 5

Mindset goal: ....
....

Eating goal: ....
....

Personal hygiene: bathe ...... teeth ......
style hair ...... get dressed ...... other ......

Pain Management Strategies:

- [ ] deep breathing
- [ ] visualization
- [ ] calming scents
- [ ] rest
- [ ] meditation
- [ ] one object focus
- [ ] PMR
- [ ] music

Something that made me smile:
....
....
Something I am proud of: ....
....
Something I am grateful for: ....
....
....
Something I am looking forward to: ....
....
....

Lowest pain level today: 1 2 3 4 5
Highest pain level today: 1 2 3 4 5

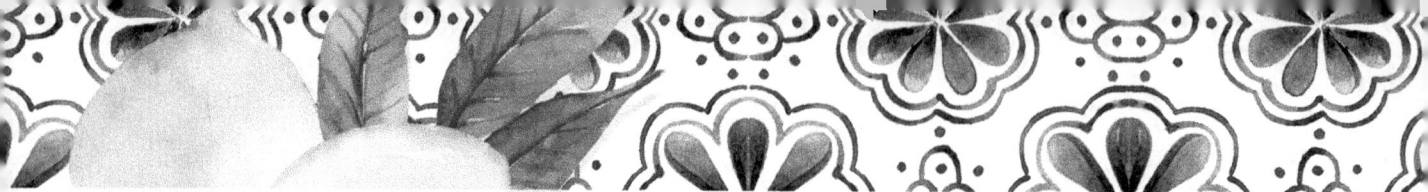

Week Fifteen

Thursday.....................

Sleep rating: 1 2 3 4 5

Mindset goal: ....
....

Eating goal: ....
....

Personal hygiene: bathe ...... teeth ......
style hair ...... get dressed ...... other ......

Pain Management Strategies:
- ☐ deep breathing ☐ meditation
- ☐ visualization ☐ one object focus
- ☐ calming scents ☐ PMR
- ☐ rest ☐ music

Something that made me smile:
....
....

Something I am proud of: ....
....

Something I am grateful for: ....
....

Something I am looking forward to: ....
....
....

Lowest pain level today: 1 2 3 4 5
Highest pain level today: 1 2 3 4 5

Friday.........................

Sleep rating: 1 2 3 4 5

Mindset goal: ....
....

Eating goal: ....
....

Personal hygiene: bathe ...... teeth ......
style hair ...... get dressed ...... other ......

Pain Management Strategies:
- ☐ deep breathing ☐ meditation
- ☐ visualization ☐ one object focus
- ☐ calming scents ☐ PMR
- ☐ rest ☐ music

Something that made me smile:
....
....

Something I am proud of: ....
....

Something I am grateful for: ....
....

Something I am looking forward to: ....
....
....

Lowest pain level today: 1 2 3 4 5
Highest pain level today: 1 2 3 4 5

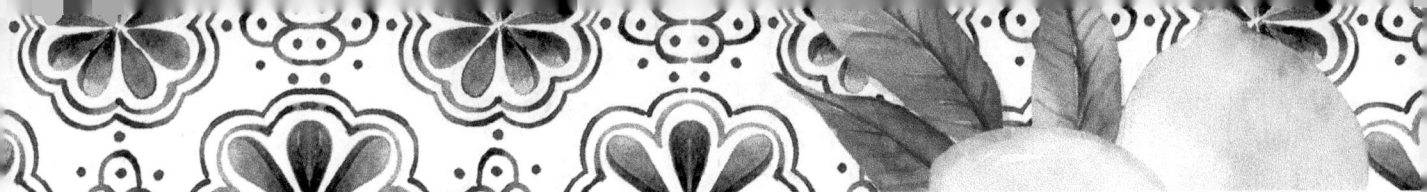

Saturday.....................

Sleep rating: 1 2 3 4 5

Mindset goal: ....
....

Eating goal: ....
....

Personal hygiene: bathe ......   teeth ......
style hair ......   get dressed ......   other ......

Pain Management Strategies:

☐ deep breathing ☐ meditation
☐ visualization ☐ one object focus
☐ calming scents ☐ PMR
☐ rest ☐ music

Something that made me smile: ....
....
....

Something I am proud of: ....
....

Something I am grateful for: ....
....
....

Something I am looking forward to: ....
....
....

Lowest pain level today: 1 2 3 4 5
Highest pain level today: 1 2 3 4 5

Sunday..........................

Sleep rating: 1 2 3 4 5

Mindset goal: ....
....

Eating goal: ....
....

Personal hygiene: bathe ......   teeth ......
style hair ......   get dressed ......   other ......

Pain Management Strategies:

☐ deep breathing ☐ meditation
☐ visualization ☐ one object focus
☐ calming scents ☐ PMR
☐ rest ☐ music

Something that made me smile: ....
....
....

Something I am proud of: ....
....

Something I am grateful for: ....
....
....

Something I am looking forward to: ....
....
....

Lowest pain level today: 1 2 3 4 5
Highest pain level today: 1 2 3 4 5

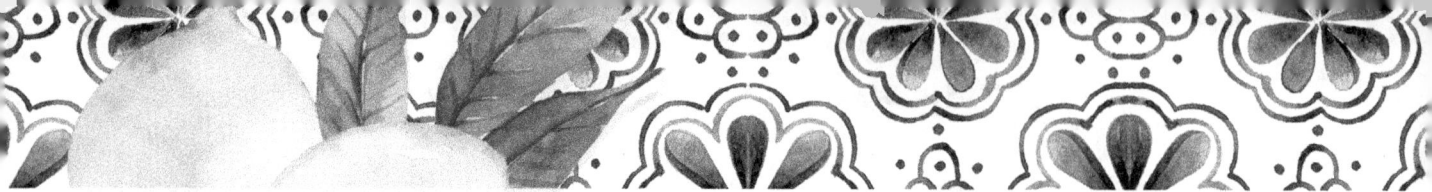

Week Sixteen

Goal for the week: ....
....

Days/Times I will leave the house or change settings: ....
....

When I will interact with friends or family: ....
....

Hobby I will work on: ....

Something new I'll try: ....

Medical tasks to do : ....
....
....

Monday...........................

Sleep rating: 1 2 3 4 5

Mindset goal: ....
....

Eating goal: ....
....

Personal hygiene: bathe ......   teeth ......
style hair ......   get dressed ......   other ......

Pain Management Strategies:

☐ deep breathing ☐ meditation
☐ visualization   ☐ one object focus
☐ calming scents ☐ PMR
☐ rest   ☐ music

Something that made me smile:
....
....
Something I am proud of: ....
....
Something I am grateful for: ....
....
Something I am looking forward to: ....
....
....
Lowest pain level today: 1 2 3 4 5
Highest pain level today: 1 2 3 4 5

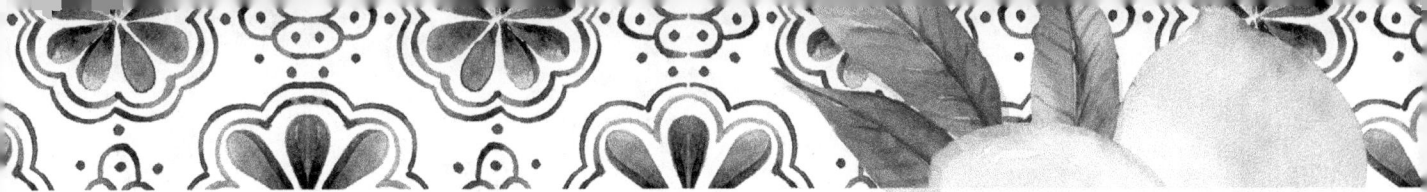

Week Sixteen

Tuesday........................

Sleep rating: 1 2 3 4 5

Mindset goal: ....
....

Eating goal: ....
....

Personal hygiene: bathe ...... teeth ......
style hair ...... get dressed ...... other ......

Pain Management Strategies:

- [ ] deep breathing
- [ ] visualization
- [ ] calming scents
- [ ] rest
- [ ] meditation
- [ ] one object focus
- [ ] PMR
- [ ] music

Something that made me smile:
....
....

Something I am proud of: ....
....

Something I am grateful for: ....
....

Something I am looking forward to: ....
....

Lowest pain level today: 1 2 3 4 5
Highest pain level today: 1 2 3 4 5

Wednesday...........................

Sleep rating: 1 2 3 4 5

Mindset goal: ....
....

Eating goal: ....
....

Personal hygiene: bathe ...... teeth ......
style hair ...... get dressed ...... other ......

Pain Management Strategies:

- [ ] deep breathing
- [ ] visualization
- [ ] calming scents
- [ ] rest
- [ ] meditation
- [ ] one object focus
- [ ] PMR
- [ ] music

Something that made me smile:
....
....

Something I am proud of: ....
....

Something I am grateful for: ....
....

Something I am looking forward to: ....
....

Lowest pain level today: 1 2 3 4 5
Highest pain level today: 1 2 3 4 5

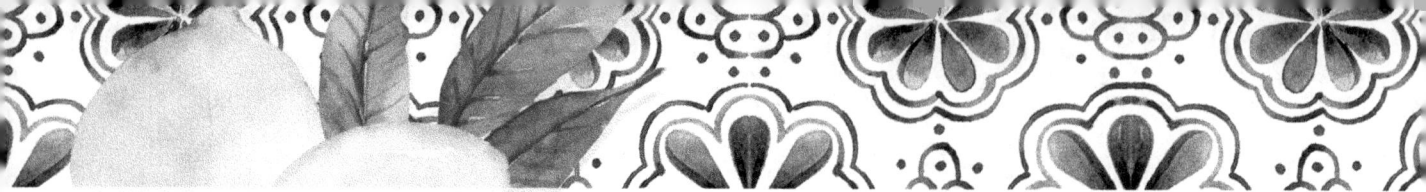

Week Sixteen

Thursday.....................

Sleep rating: 1 2 3 4 5

Mindset goal: ....
....

Eating goal: ....
....

Personal hygiene: bathe ......   teeth ......
style hair ......   get dressed ......   other ......

Pain Management Strategies:

☐ deep breathing ☐ meditation
☐ visualization ☐ one object focus
☐ calming scents ☐ PMR
☐ rest ☐ music

Something that made me smile:
....
....
Something I am proud of: ....
....
Something I am grateful for: ....
....
Something I am looking forward to: ....
....
....

Lowest pain level today: 1 2 3 4 5
Highest pain level today: 1 2 3 4 5

Friday...........................

Sleep rating: 1 2 3 4 5

Mindset goal: ....
....

Eating goal: ....
....

Personal hygiene: bathe ......   teeth ......
style hair ......   get dressed ......   other ......

Pain Management Strategies:

☐ deep breathing ☐ meditation
☐ visualization ☐ one object focus
☐ calming scents ☐ PMR
☐ rest ☐ music

Something that made me smile:
....
....
Something I am proud of: ....
....
Something I am grateful for: ....
....
Something I am looking forward to: ....
....
....

Lowest pain level today: 1 2 3 4 5
Highest pain level today: 1 2 3 4 5

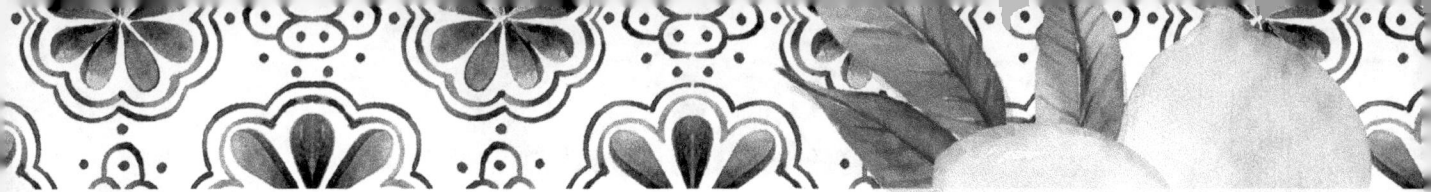

Week Sixteen

Saturday.....................

Sleep rating: 1 2 3 4 5

Mindset goal: ....
....

Eating goal: ....
....

Personal hygiene: bathe ...... teeth ......
style hair ...... get dressed ...... other ......

Pain Management Strategies:

☐ deep breathing ☐ meditation
☐ visualization ☐ one object focus
☐ calming scents ☐ PMR
☐ rest ☐ music

Something that made me smile:
....
....
Something I am proud of: ....
....
....
Something I am grateful for: ....
....
....
Something I am looking forward to: ....
....
....
Lowest pain level today: 1 2 3 4 5
Highest pain level today: 1 2 3 4 5

Sunday........................

Sleep rating: 1 2 3 4 5

Mindset goal: ....
....

Eating goal: ....
....

Personal hygiene: bathe ...... teeth ......
style hair ...... get dressed ...... other ......

Pain Management Strategies:

☐ deep breathing ☐ meditation
☐ visualization ☐ one object focus
☐ calming scents ☐ PMR
☐ rest ☐ music

Something that made me smile:
....
....
Something I am proud of: ....
....
....
Something I am grateful for: ....
....
....
Something I am looking forward to: ....
....
....
Lowest pain level today: 1 2 3 4 5
Highest pain level today: 1 2 3 4 5

Monthly Reflection

Happy Distraction

Draw the other half of these crystals. No pressure! Just have fun.

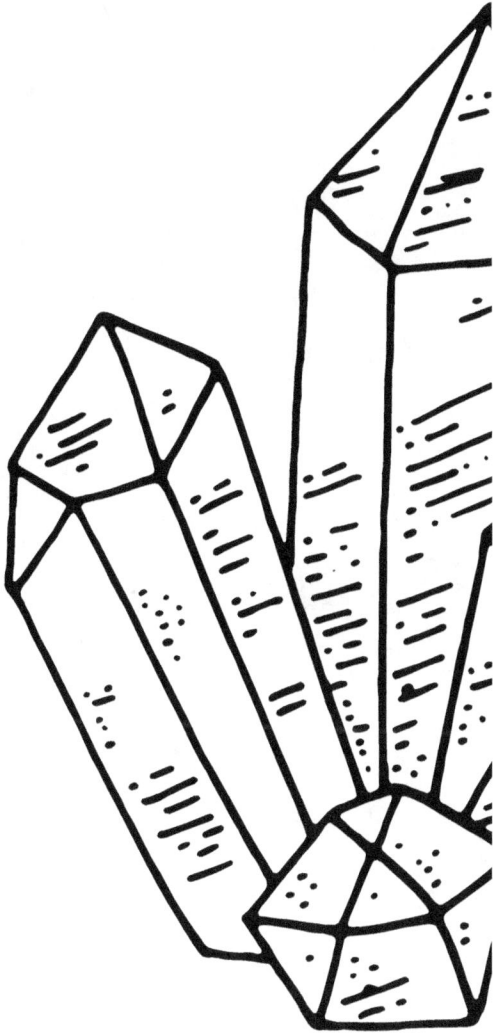

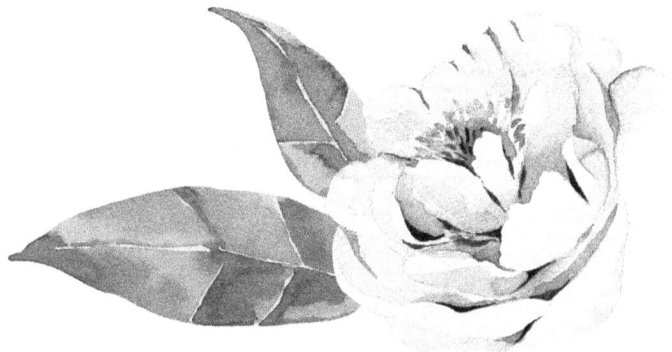

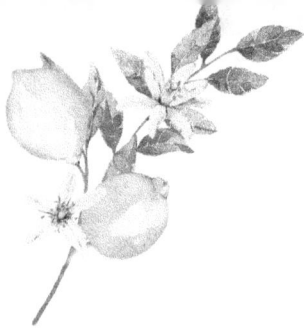

Week Seventeen

Goal for the week: ....
....

Days/Times I will leave the house or change settings: ....
....

When I will interact with friends or family: ....
....

Hobby I will work on: ....

Something new I'll try: ....

Medical tasks to do : ....
....
....

Monday.......................

Sleep rating: 1   2   3   4   5

Mindset goal: ....
....

Eating goal: ....
....

Personal hygiene: bathe ......   teeth ......
style hair ......   get dressed ......   other ......

Pain Management Strategies:

☐ deep breathing ☐ meditation
☐ visualization ☐ one object focus
☐ calming scents ☐ PMR
☐ rest ☐ music

Something that made me smile:
....
....
Something I am proud of: ....
....
Something I am grateful for: ....
....
....
Something I am looking forward to: ....
....
....
Lowest pain level today: 1 2 3 4 5
Highest pain level today: 1 2 3 4 5

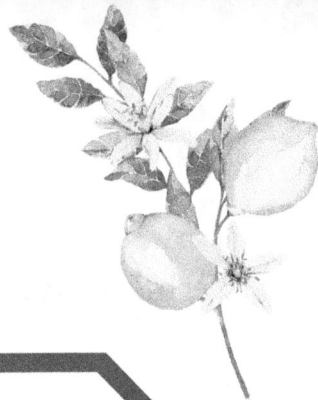

Week Seventeen

Tuesday...................

Sleep rating: 1 2 3 4 5

Mindset goal: ....
....

Eating goal: ....
....

Personal hygiene: bathe ...... teeth ......
style hair ...... get dressed ...... other ......

Pain Management Strategies:

☐ deep breathing ☐ meditation
☐ visualization ☐ one object focus
☐ calming scents ☐ PMR
☐ rest ☐ music

Something that made me smile:
....
....
Something I am proud of: ....
....
Something I am grateful for: ....
....
Something I am looking forward to: ....
....
....

Lowest pain level today: 1 2 3 4 5
Highest pain level today: 1 2 3 4 5

Wednesday.........................

Sleep rating: 1 2 3 4 5

Mindset goal: ....
....

Eating goal: ....
....

Personal hygiene: bathe ...... teeth ......
style hair ...... get dressed ...... other ......

Pain Management Strategies:

☐ deep breathing ☐ meditation
☐ visualization ☐ one object focus
☐ calming scents ☐ PMR
☐ rest ☐ music

Something that made me smile:
....
....
Something I am proud of: ....
....
Something I am grateful for: ....
....
....
Something I am looking forward to: ....
....
....

Lowest pain level today: 1 2 3 4 5
Highest pain level today: 1 2 3 4 5

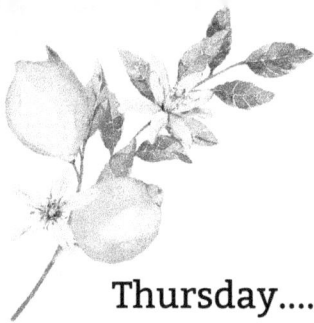

Sleep rating: 1 2 3 4 5

Mindset goal: ....
....

Eating goal: ....
....

Personal hygiene: bathe ......   teeth ......
style hair ......   get dressed ......   other ......

Pain Management Strategies:

- [ ] deep breathing [ ] meditation
- [ ] visualization [ ] one object focus
- [ ] calming scents [ ] PMR
- [ ] rest [ ] music

Something that made me smile:
....
....

Something I am proud of: ....
....

Something I am grateful for: ....
....

Something I am looking forward to: ....
....
....

Lowest pain level today: 1 2 3 4 5
Highest pain level today: 1 2 3 4 5

Friday........................

Sleep rating: 1 2 3 4 5

Mindset goal: ....
....

Eating goal: ....
....

Personal hygiene: bathe ......   teeth ......
style hair ......   get dressed ......   other ......

Pain Management Strategies:

- [ ] deep breathing [ ] meditation
- [ ] visualization [ ] one object focus
- [ ] calming scents [ ] PMR
- [ ] rest [ ] music

Something that made me smile:
....
....

Something I am proud of: ....
....

Something I am grateful for: ....
....

Something I am looking forward to: ....
....
....

Lowest pain level today: 1 2 3 4 5
Highest pain level today: 1 2 3 4 5

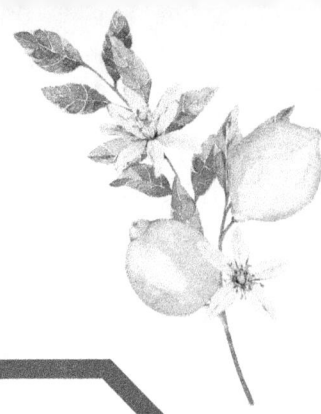

Week Seventeen

Saturday......................

Sleep rating: 1 2 3 4 5

Mindset goal: ....

....

Eating goal: ....

....

Personal hygiene: bathe ...... teeth ......
style hair ...... get dressed ...... other ......

Pain Management Strategies:

☐ deep breathing ☐ meditation
☐ visualization   ☐ one object focus
☐ calming scents ☐ PMR
☐ rest   ☐ music

Something that made me smile:

....

....

Something I am proud of: ....

....

Something I am grateful for: ....

....

Something I am looking forward to: ....

....

Lowest pain level today: 1 2 3 4 5
Highest pain level today: 1 2 3 4 5

Sunday........................

Sleep rating: 1 2 3 4 5

Mindset goal: ....

....

Eating goal: ....

....

Personal hygiene: bathe ...... teeth ......
style hair ...... get dressed ...... other ......

Pain Management Strategies:

☐ deep breathing ☐ meditation
☐ visualization   ☐ one object focus
☐ calming scents ☐ PMR
☐ rest   ☐ music

Something that made me smile:

....

....

Something I am proud of: ....

....

Something I am grateful for: ....

....

Something I am looking forward to: ....

....

Lowest pain level today: 1 2 3 4 5
Highest pain level today: 1 2 3 4 5

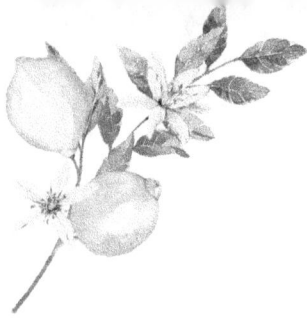

Week Eighteen

Goal for the week: ....
....

Days/Times I will leave the house or change settings: ....
....

When I will interact with friends or family: ....
....

Hobby I will work on: ....

Something new I'll try: ....

Medical tasks to do : ....
....
....

Monday.......................

Sleep rating: 1 2 3 4 5

Mindset goal: ....
....

Eating goal: ....
....

Personal hygiene: bathe ......   teeth ......
style hair ......   get dressed ......   other ......

Pain Management Strategies:

- [ ] deep breathing [ ] meditation
- [ ] visualization   [ ] one object focus
- [ ] calming scents [ ] PMR
- [ ] rest   [ ] music

Something that made me smile:
....
....

Something I am proud of: ....
....

Something I am grateful for: ....
....

Something I am looking forward to: ....
....

Lowest pain level today: 1 2 3 4 5
Highest pain level today: 1 2 3 4 5

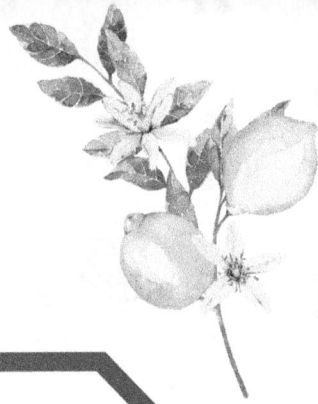

Week Eighteen

Tuesday..........................

Sleep rating: 1 2 3 4 5

Mindset goal: ....

....

Eating goal: ....

....

Personal hygiene: bathe ...... teeth ......
style hair ...... get dressed ...... other ......

Pain Management Strategies:

☐ deep breathing   ☐ meditation
☐ visualization   ☐ one object focus
☐ calming scents   ☐ PMR
☐ rest   ☐ music

Something that made me smile:

....

....

Something I am proud of: ....

....

Something I am grateful for: ....

....

Something I am looking forward to: ....

....

....

Lowest pain level today: 1 2 3 4 5
Highest pain level today: 1 2 3 4 5

Wednesday...........................

Sleep rating: 1 2 3 4 5

Mindset goal: ....

....

Eating goal: ....

....

Personal hygiene: bathe ...... teeth ......
style hair ...... get dressed ...... other ......

Pain Management Strategies:

☐ deep breathing   ☐ meditation
☐ visualization   ☐ one object focus
☐ calming scents   ☐ PMR
☐ rest   ☐ music

Something that made me smile:

....

....

Something I am proud of: ....

....

Something I am grateful for: ....

....

....

Something I am looking forward to: ....

....

....

Lowest pain level today: 1 2 3 4 5
Highest pain level today: 1 2 3 4 5

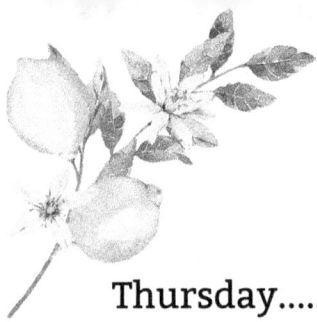

Sleep rating: 1 2 3 4 5

Mindset goal: ....
....

Eating goal: ....
....

Personal hygiene: bathe ......   teeth ......
style hair ......   get dressed ......   other ......

Pain Management Strategies:

☐ deep breathing   ☐ meditation
☐ visualization   ☐ one object focus
☐ calming scents   ☐ PMR
☐ rest   ☐ music

Something that made me smile:
....
....

Something I am proud of: ....
....

Something I am grateful for: ....
....

Something I am looking forward to: ....
....
....

Lowest pain level today: 1 2 3 4 5
Highest pain level today: 1 2 3 4 5

Friday........................

Sleep rating: 1 2 3 4 5

Mindset goal: ....
....

Eating goal: ....
....

Personal hygiene: bathe ......   teeth ......
style hair ......   get dressed ......   other ......

Pain Management Strategies:

☐ deep breathing   ☐ meditation
☐ visualization   ☐ one object focus
☐ calming scents   ☐ PMR
☐ rest   ☐ music

Something that made me smile:
....
....

Something I am proud of: ....
....

Something I am grateful for: ....
....

Something I am looking forward to: ....
....
....

Lowest pain level today: 1 2 3 4 5
Highest pain level today: 1 2 3 4 5

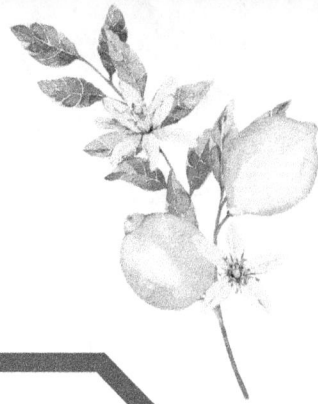

Week Eighteen

Saturday.....................

Sleep rating: 1 2 3 4 5

Mindset goal: ....
....

Eating goal: ....
....

Personal hygiene: bathe ...... teeth ......
style hair ...... get dressed ...... other ......

Pain Management Strategies:

☐ deep breathing ☐ meditation
☐ visualization ☐ one object focus
☐ calming scents ☐ PMR
☐ rest ☐ music

Something that made me smile:
....
....
Something I am proud of: ....
....
Something I am grateful for: ....
....
Something I am looking forward to: ....
....
....
Lowest pain level today: 1 2 3 4 5
Highest pain level today: 1 2 3 4 5

Sunday........................

Sleep rating: 1 2 3 4 5

Mindset goal: ....
....

Eating goal: ....
....

Personal hygiene: bathe ...... teeth ......
style hair ...... get dressed ...... other ......

Pain Management Strategies:

☐ deep breathing ☐ meditation
☐ visualization ☐ one object focus
☐ calming scents ☐ PMR
☐ rest ☐ music

Something that made me smile:
....
....
Something I am proud of: ....
....
Something I am grateful for: ....
....
Something I am looking forward to: ....
....
....
Lowest pain level today: 1 2 3 4 5
Highest pain level today: 1 2 3 4 5

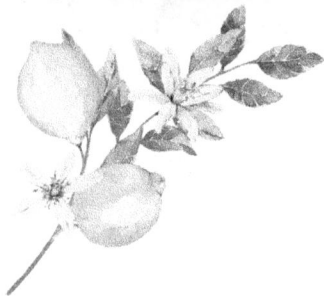

Week Nineteen

Goal for the week: ....

....

Days/Times I will leave the house or change settings: ....

....

When I will interact with friends or family: ....

....

Hobby I will work on: ....

Something new I'll try: ....

Medical tasks to do : ....

....

....

Monday........................

Sleep rating: 1   2   3   4   5

Mindset goal: ....

....

Eating goal: ....

....

Personal hygiene: bathe ...... teeth ......
style hair ......   get dressed ......   other ......

Pain Management Strategies:

- [ ] deep breathing
- [ ] visualization
- [ ] calming scents
- [ ] rest
- [ ] meditation
- [ ] one object focus
- [ ] PMR
- [ ] music

Something that made me smile:

....

....

Something I am proud of: ....

....

Something I am grateful for: ....

....

....

Something I am looking forward to: ....

....

....

Lowest pain level today: 1 2 3 4 5
Highest pain level today: 1 2 3 4 5

Week Nineteen

Tuesday...........................

Sleep rating: 1 2 3 4 5

Mindset goal: ....
....

Eating goal: ....
....

Personal hygiene: bathe ......   teeth ......
style hair ......   get dressed ......   other ......

Pain Management Strategies:

☐ deep breathing ☐ meditation
☐ visualization ☐ one object focus
☐ calming scents ☐ PMR
☐ rest ☐ music

Something that made me smile:
....
....
Something I am proud of: ....
....
Something I am grateful for: ....
....
Something I am looking forward to: ....
....
....
Lowest pain level today: 1 2 3 4 5
Highest pain level today: 1 2 3 4 5

Wednesday...........................

Sleep rating: 1 2 3 4 5

Mindset goal: ....
....

Eating goal: ....
....

Personal hygiene: bathe ......   teeth ......
style hair ......   get dressed ......   other ......

Pain Management Strategies:

☐ deep breathing ☐ meditation
☐ visualization ☐ one object focus
☐ calming scents ☐ PMR
☐ rest ☐ music

Something that made me smile:
....
....
Something I am proud of: ....
....
Something I am grateful for: ....
....
Something I am looking forward to: ....
....
....
Lowest pain level today: 1 2 3 4 5
Highest pain level today: 1 2 3 4 5

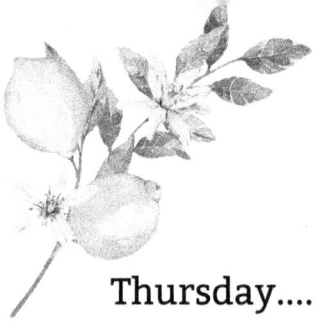

Week Nineteen

Thursday..................

Sleep rating: 1 2 3 4 5

Mindset goal: ....
....

Eating goal: ....
....

Personal hygiene: bathe ...... teeth ......
style hair ...... get dressed ...... other ......

Pain Management Strategies:

- [ ] deep breathing
- [ ] visualization
- [ ] calming scents
- [ ] rest
- [ ] meditation
- [ ] one object focus
- [ ] PMR
- [ ] music

Something that made me smile:
....
....

Something I am proud of: ....
....

Something I am grateful for: ....
....

Something I am looking forward to: ....
....

Lowest pain level today: 1 2 3 4 5
Highest pain level today: 1 2 3 4 5

Friday.......................

Sleep rating: 1 2 3 4 5

Mindset goal: ....
....

Eating goal: ....
....

Personal hygiene: bathe ...... teeth ......
style hair ...... get dressed ...... other ......

Pain Management Strategies:

- [ ] deep breathing
- [ ] visualization
- [ ] calming scents
- [ ] rest
- [ ] meditation
- [ ] one object focus
- [ ] PMR
- [ ] music

Something that made me smile:
....
....

Something I am proud of: ....
....

Something I am grateful for: ....
....

Something I am looking forward to: ....
....

Lowest pain level today: 1 2 3 4 5
Highest pain level today: 1 2 3 4 5

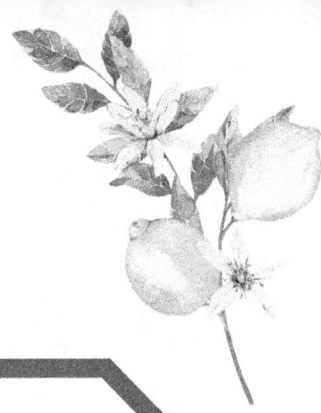

Saturday.....................

Sleep rating: 1 2 3 4 5

Mindset goal: ....
....

Eating goal: ....
....

Personal hygiene: bathe ......   teeth ......
style hair ......   get dressed ......   other ......

Pain Management Strategies:

☐ deep breathing ☐ meditation
☐ visualization ☐ one object focus
☐ calming scents ☐ PMR
☐ rest ☐ music

Something that made me smile:
....
....
Something I am proud of: ....
....
Something I am grateful for: ....
....
Something I am looking forward to: ....
....
....

Lowest pain level today: 1 2 3 4 5
Highest pain level today: 1 2 3 4 5

Sunday........................

Sleep rating: 1 2 3 4 5

Mindset goal: ....
....

Eating goal: ....
....

Personal hygiene: bathe ......   teeth ......
style hair ......   get dressed ......   other ......

Pain Management Strategies:

☐ deep breathing ☐ meditation
☐ visualization ☐ one object focus
☐ calming scents ☐ PMR
☐ rest ☐ music

Something that made me smile:
....
....
Something I am proud of: ....
....
Something I am grateful for: ....
....
....
Something I am looking forward to: ....
....
....

Lowest pain level today: 1 2 3 4 5
Highest pain level today: 1 2 3 4 5

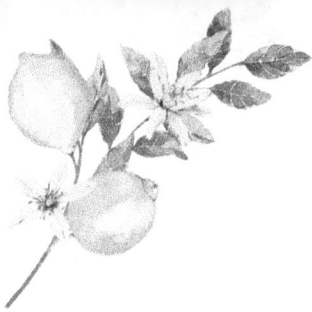

Week Twenty

Goal for the week: ....
....

Days/Times I will leave the house or change settings: ....
....

When I will interact with friends or family: ....
....

Hobby I will work on: ....

Something new I'll try: ....

Medical tasks to do : ....
....
....

Monday.........................

Sleep rating: 1 2 3 4 5

Mindset goal: ....
....

Eating goal: ....
....

Personal hygiene: bathe ......   teeth ......
style hair ......   get dressed ......   other ......

Pain Management Strategies:

- [ ] deep breathing [ ] meditation
- [ ] visualization [ ] one object focus
- [ ] calming scents [ ] PMR
- [ ] rest [ ] music

Something that made me smile:
....
....

Something I am proud of: ....
....

Something I am grateful for: ....
....

Something I am looking forward to: ....
....
....

Lowest pain level today: 1 2 3 4 5
Highest pain level today: 1 2 3 4 5

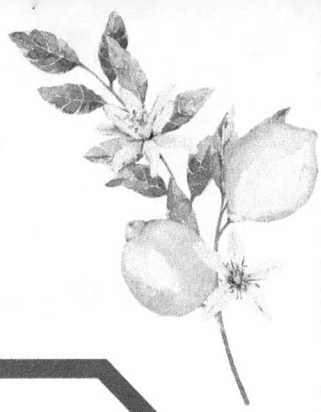

Week Twenty

Tuesday..........................

Sleep rating: 1 2 3 4 5

Mindset goal: ....
....

Eating goal: ....
....

Personal hygiene: bathe ...... teeth ......
style hair ...... get dressed ...... other ......

Pain Management Strategies:

☐ deep breathing ☐ meditation
☐ visualization ☐ one object focus
☐ calming scents ☐ PMR
☐ rest ☐ music

Something that made me smile:
....
....
Something I am proud of: ....
....
Something I am grateful for: ....
....
Something I am looking forward to: ....
....
....
Lowest pain level today: 1 2 3 4 5
Highest pain level today: 1 2 3 4 5

Wednesday..........................

Sleep rating: 1 2 3 4 5

Mindset goal: ....
....

Eating goal: ....
....

Personal hygiene: bathe ...... teeth ......
style hair ...... get dressed ...... other ......

Pain Management Strategies:

☐ deep breathing ☐ meditation
☐ visualization ☐ one object focus
☐ calming scents ☐ PMR
☐ rest ☐ music

Something that made me smile:
....
....
Something I am proud of: ....
....
Something I am grateful for: ....
....
Something I am looking forward to: ....
....
....
Lowest pain level today: 1 2 3 4 5
Highest pain level today: 1 2 3 4 5

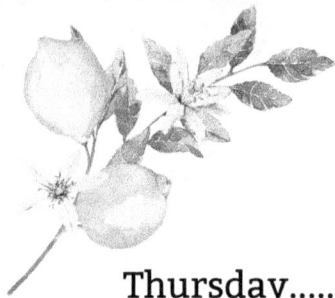

Thursday..................... *Week Twenty*

Sleep rating: 1 2 3 4 5

Mindset goal: ....
....

Eating goal: ....
....

Personal hygiene: bathe ......   teeth ......
style hair ......   get dressed ......   other ......

Pain Management Strategies:

☐ deep breathing ☐ meditation
☐ visualization   ☐ one object focus
☐ calming scents ☐ PMR
☐ rest   ☐ music

Something that made me smile:
....
....
Something I am proud of: ....
....
Something I am grateful for: ....
....
Something I am looking forward to: ....
....
....

Lowest pain level today: 1 2 3 4 5
Highest pain level today: 1 2 3 4 5

Friday........................

Sleep rating: 1 2 3 4 5

Mindset goal: ....
....

Eating goal: ....
....

Personal hygiene: bathe ......   teeth ......
style hair ......   get dressed ......   other ......

Pain Management Strategies:

☐ deep breathing ☐ meditation
☐ visualization   ☐ one object focus
☐ calming scents ☐ PMR
☐ rest   ☐ music

Something that made me smile:
....
....
Something I am proud of: ....
....
Something I am grateful for: ....
....
Something I am looking forward to: ....
....
....

Lowest pain level today: 1 2 3 4 5
Highest pain level today: 1 2 3 4 5

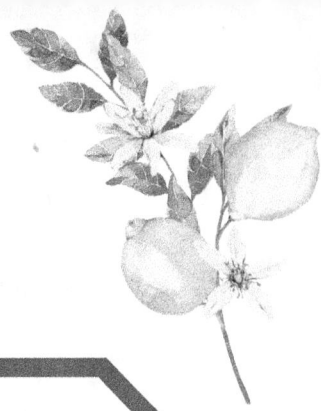

Saturday........................ *Week Twenty*

Sleep rating: 1 2 3 4 5

Mindset goal: ....
....

Eating goal: ....
....

Personal hygiene: bathe ...... teeth ......
style hair ...... get dressed ...... other ......

Pain Management Strategies:

- ☐ deep breathing ☐ meditation
- ☐ visualization ☐ one object focus
- ☐ calming scents ☐ PMR
- ☐ rest ☐ music

Something that made me smile:
....
....

Something I am proud of: ....
....

Something I am grateful for: ....
....

Something I am looking forward to: ....
....

Lowest pain level today: 1 2 3 4 5
Highest pain level today: 1 2 3 4 5

Sunday........................

Sleep rating: 1 2 3 4 5

Mindset goal: ....
....

Eating goal: ....
....

Personal hygiene: bathe ...... teeth ......
style hair ...... get dressed ...... other ......

Pain Management Strategies:

- ☐ deep breathing ☐ meditation
- ☐ visualization ☐ one object focus
- ☐ calming scents ☐ PMR
- ☐ rest ☐ music

Something that made me smile:
....
....

Something I am proud of: ....
....

Something I am grateful for: ....
....

Something I am looking forward to: ....
....

Lowest pain level today: 1 2 3 4 5
Highest pain level today: 1 2 3 4 5

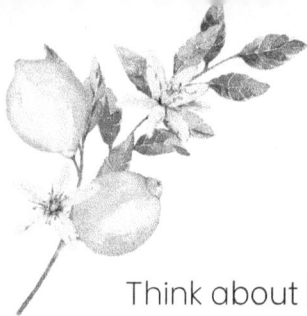

Monthly Reflection

Think about how your mental health was this month. Did you use the strategies?
When were you your best? Your worst?

....

....

....

....

....

....

....

....

....

....

....

....

....

....

....

....

....

....

....

Happy Distraction

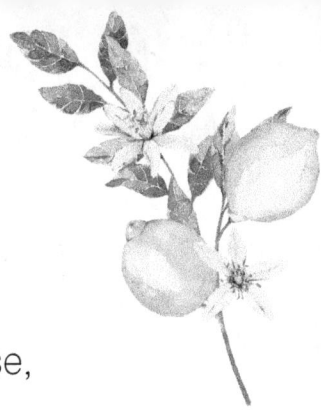

Word sandwich: Find the word that goes in the middle. It will be the second half of the first phrase, and the first half of the second phrase.

Example: apple _(pie)_ chart

dog...arrest

snow...hole

cross...side

bread...sharpener

cruise...tower

sunshine..fair

paper...board

seat...sander

chicken...implant

hot...leash

cup...walk

jingle...................................south

dish...................................scum

passing.......................................bryant

rest...sign

friend................................wreck

cold...study

black...................................glasses

hot...protector

fortune...................................miles

note...keeper

rat...car

candy...husk

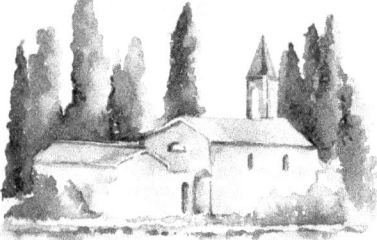

Week Twenty-One

Goal for the week: ....
....

Days/Times I will leave the house or change settings: ....
....

When I will interact with friends or family: ....
....

Hobby I will work on: ....

Something new I'll try: ....

Medical tasks to do : ....
....
....

Monday........................

Sleep rating: 1 2 3 4 5

Mindset goal: ....
....

Eating goal: ....
....

Personal hygiene: bathe ...... teeth ......
style hair ...... get dressed ...... other ......

Pain Management Strategies:

- [ ] deep breathing [ ] meditation
- [ ] visualization [ ] one object focus
- [ ] calming scents [ ] PMR
- [ ] rest [ ] music

Something that made me smile:
....
....
Something I am proud of: ....
....
Something I am grateful for: ....
....
Something I am looking forward to: ....
....
....

Lowest pain level today: 1 2 3 4 5
Highest pain level today: 1 2 3 4 5

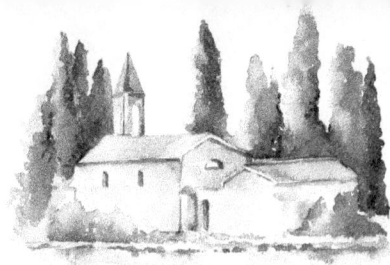

Week Twenty=One

Tuesday......................

Sleep rating: 1 2 3 4 5

Mindset goal: ....
....

Eating goal: ....
....

Personal hygiene: bathe ...... teeth ......
style hair ...... get dressed ...... other ......

Pain Management Strategies:

☐ deep breathing ☐ meditation
☐ visualization ☐ one object focus
☐ calming scents ☐ PMR
☐ rest ☐ music

Something that made me smile:
....
....

Something I am proud of: ....
....

Something I am grateful for: ....
....

Something I am looking forward to: ....
....

Lowest pain level today: 1 2 3 4 5
Highest pain level today: 1 2 3 4 5

Wednesday........................

Sleep rating: 1 2 3 4 5

Mindset goal: ....
....

Eating goal: ....
....

Personal hygiene: bathe ...... teeth ......
style hair ...... get dressed ...... other ......

Pain Management Strategies:

☐ deep breathing ☐ meditation
☐ visualization ☐ one object focus
☐ calming scents ☐ PMR
☐ rest ☐ music

Something that made me smile:
....
....

Something I am proud of: ....
....

Something I am grateful for: ....
....

Something I am looking forward to: ....
....

Lowest pain level today: 1 2 3 4 5
Highest pain level today: 1 2 3 4 5

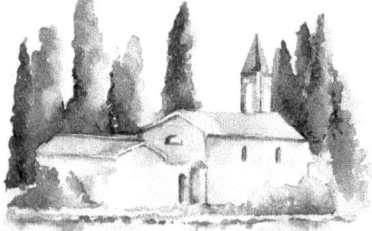

Week Twenty-One

Thursday.....................

Sleep rating: 1 2 3 4 5

Mindset goal: ....
....

Eating goal: ....
....

Personal hygiene: bathe ......   teeth ......
style hair ......   get dressed ......   other ......

Pain Management Strategies:

☐ deep breathing   ☐ meditation
☐ visualization   ☐ one object focus
☐ calming scents   ☐ PMR
☐ rest   ☐ music

Something that made me smile:
....
....

Something I am proud of: ....
....

Something I am grateful for: ....
....

Something I am looking forward to: ....
....
....

Lowest pain level today: 1 2 3 4 5
Highest pain level today: 1 2 3 4 5

Friday.........................

Sleep rating: 1 2 3 4 5

Mindset goal: ....
....

Eating goal: ....
....

Personal hygiene: bathe ......   teeth ......
style hair ......   get dressed ......   other ......

Pain Management Strategies:

☐ deep breathing   ☐ meditation
☐ visualization   ☐ one object focus
☐ calming scents   ☐ PMR
☐ rest   ☐ music

Something that made me smile:
....
....

Something I am proud of: ....
....

Something I am grateful for: ....
....

Something I am looking forward to: ....
....
....

Lowest pain level today: 1 2 3 4 5
Highest pain level today: 1 2 3 4 5

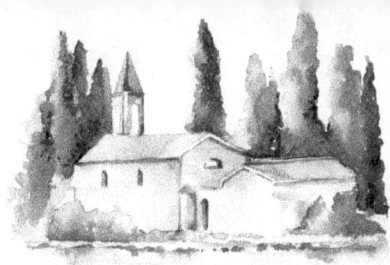

Saturday...................

Sleep rating: 1 2 3 4 5

Mindset goal: ....
....

Eating goal: ....
....

Personal hygiene: bathe ...... teeth ......
style hair ...... get dressed ...... other ......

Pain Management Strategies:

- [ ] deep breathing
- [ ] visualization
- [ ] calming scents
- [ ] rest
- [ ] meditation
- [ ] one object focus
- [ ] PMR
- [ ] music

Something that made me smile:
....
....

Something I am proud of: ....
....

Something I am grateful for: ....
....

Something I am looking forward to: ....
....

Lowest pain level today: 1 2 3 4 5
Highest pain level today: 1 2 3 4 5

Sunday.........................

Sleep rating: 1 2 3 4 5

Mindset goal: ....
....

Eating goal: ....
....

Personal hygiene: bathe ...... teeth ......
style hair ...... get dressed ...... other ......

Pain Management Strategies:

- [ ] deep breathing
- [ ] visualization
- [ ] calming scents
- [ ] rest
- [ ] meditation
- [ ] one object focus
- [ ] PMR
- [ ] music

Something that made me smile:
....
....

Something I am proud of: ....
....

Something I am grateful for: ....
....

Something I am looking forward to: ....
....

Lowest pain level today: 1 2 3 4 5
Highest pain level today: 1 2 3 4 5

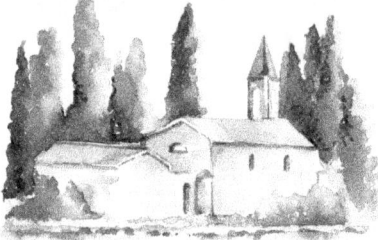

Week Twenty-Two

Goal for the week: ....
....

Days/Times I will leave the house or change settings: ....
....

When I will interact with friends or family: ....
....

Hobby I will work on: ....

Something new I'll try: ....

Medical tasks to do : ....
....
....

Monday........................

Sleep rating: 1 2 3 4 5

Mindset goal: ....
....

Eating goal: ....
....

Personal hygiene: bathe ......   teeth ......
style hair ......   get dressed ......   other ......

Pain Management Strategies:

☐ deep breathing ☐ meditation
☐ visualization   ☐ one object focus
☐ calming scents ☐ PMR
☐ rest   ☐ music

Something that made me smile:
....
....
Something I am proud of: ....
....
Something I am grateful for: ....
....
Something I am looking forward to: ....
....
....
Lowest pain level today: 1 2 3 4 5
Highest pain level today: 1 2 3 4 5

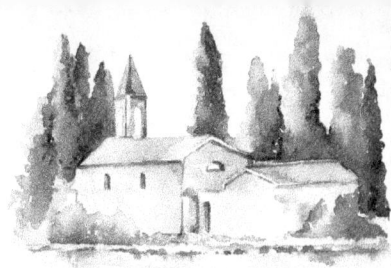

Week Twenty-Two

Tuesday..........................

Sleep rating: 1 2 3 4 5

Mindset goal: ....
....

Eating goal: ....
....

Personal hygiene: bathe ......   teeth ......
style hair ......   get dressed ......   other ......

Pain Management Strategies:

☐ deep breathing ☐ meditation
☐ visualization   ☐ one object focus
☐ calming scents ☐ PMR
☐ rest   ☐ music

Something that made me smile:
....
....
Something I am proud of: ....
....
Something I am grateful for: ....
....
Something I am looking forward to: ....
....
....

Lowest pain level today: 1 2 3 4 5
Highest pain level today: 1 2 3 4 5

Wednesday..........................

Sleep rating: 1 2 3 4 5

Mindset goal: ....
....

Eating goal: ....
....

Personal hygiene: bathe ......   teeth ......
style hair ......   get dressed ......   other ......

Pain Management Strategies:

☐ deep breathing ☐ meditation
☐ visualization   ☐ one object focus
☐ calming scents ☐ PMR
☐ rest   ☐ music

Something that made me smile:
....
....
Something I am proud of: ....
....
Something I am grateful for: ....
....
Something I am looking forward to: ....
....
....

Lowest pain level today: 1 2 3 4 5
Highest pain level today: 1 2 3 4 5

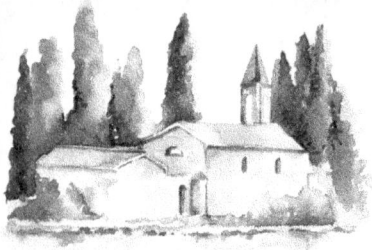

Sleep rating: 1 2 3 4 5

Mindset goal: ....
....

Eating goal: ....
....

Personal hygiene: bathe ...... teeth ......
style hair ...... get dressed ...... other ......

Pain Management Strategies:

☐ deep breathing ☐ meditation
☐ visualization ☐ one object focus
☐ calming scents ☐ PMR
☐ rest ☐ music

Something that made me smile:
....
....
Something I am proud of: ....
....
Something I am grateful for: ....
....
Something I am looking forward to: ....
....
....
Lowest pain level today: 1 2 3 4 5
Highest pain level today: 1 2 3 4 5

Friday..........................

Sleep rating: 1 2 3 4 5

Mindset goal: ....
....

Eating goal: ....
....

Personal hygiene: bathe ...... teeth ......
style hair ...... get dressed ...... other ......

Pain Management Strategies:

☐ deep breathing ☐ meditation
☐ visualization ☐ one object focus
☐ calming scents ☐ PMR
☐ rest ☐ music

Something that made me smile:
....
....
Something I am proud of: ....
....
Something I am grateful for: ....
....
Something I am looking forward to: ....
....
....
Lowest pain level today: 1 2 3 4 5
Highest pain level today: 1 2 3 4 5

Saturday......................

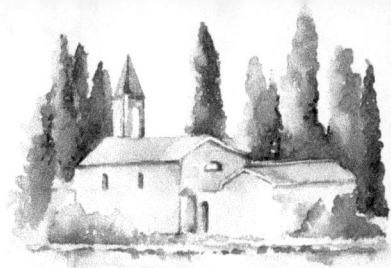

Week Twenty-Two

Sleep rating: 1 2 3 4 5

Mindset goal: ....
....

Eating goal: ....
....

Personal hygiene: bathe ......   teeth ......
style hair ......   get dressed ......   other ......

Pain Management Strategies:

☐ deep breathing ☐ meditation
☐ visualization ☐ one object focus
☐ calming scents ☐ PMR
☐ rest ☐ music

Something that made me smile:
....
....
Something I am proud of: ....
....
Something I am grateful for: ....
....
Something I am looking forward to: ....
....
....
Lowest pain level today: 1 2 3 4 5
Highest pain level today: 1 2 3 4 5

Sunday.........................

Sleep rating: 1 2 3 4 5

Mindset goal: ....
....

Eating goal: ....
....

Personal hygiene: bathe ......   teeth ......
style hair ......   get dressed ......   other ......

Pain Management Strategies:

☐ deep breathing ☐ meditation
☐ visualization ☐ one object focus
☐ calming scents ☐ PMR
☐ rest ☐ music

Something that made me smile:
....
....
Something I am proud of: ....
....
Something I am grateful for: ....
....
....
Something I am looking forward to: ....
....
....
Lowest pain level today: 1 2 3 4 5
Highest pain level today: 1 2 3 4 5

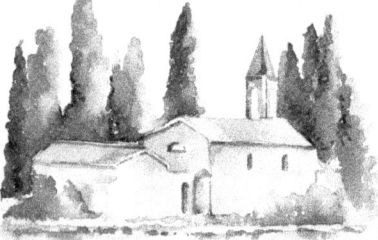

Week Twenty-Three

Goal for the week: ....
....

Days/Times I will leave the house or change settings: ....
....

When I will interact with friends or family: ....
....

Hobby I will work on: ....

Something new I'll try: ....

Medical tasks to do : ....
....
....

Monday.........................

Sleep rating: 1 2 3 4 5

Mindset goal: ....
....

Eating goal: ....
....

Personal hygiene: bathe ......   teeth ......
style hair ......   get dressed ......   other ......

Pain Management Strategies:

☐ deep breathing ☐ meditation
☐ visualization ☐ one object focus
☐ calming scents ☐ PMR
☐ rest ☐ music

Something that made me smile:
....
....
Something I am proud of: ....
....
Something I am grateful for: ....
....
Something I am looking forward to: ....
....
....
Lowest pain level today: 1 2 3 4 5
Highest pain level today: 1 2 3 4 5

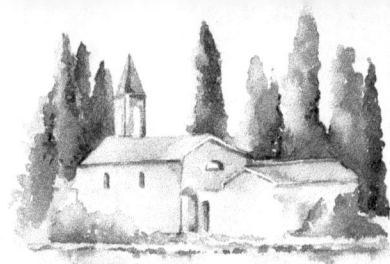

Sleep rating: 1 2 3 4 5

Mindset goal: ....
....

Eating goal: ....
....

Personal hygiene: bathe ...... teeth ......
style hair ...... get dressed ...... other ......

Pain Management Strategies:

☐ deep breathing ☐ meditation
☐ visualization ☐ one object focus
☐ calming scents ☐ PMR
☐ rest ☐ music

Something that made me smile:
....
....

Something I am proud of: ....
....

Something I am grateful for: ....
....

Something I am looking forward to: ....
....

Lowest pain level today: 1 2 3 4 5
Highest pain level today: 1 2 3 4 5

Wednesday.........................

Sleep rating: 1 2 3 4 5

Mindset goal: ....
....

Eating goal: ....
....

Personal hygiene: bathe ...... teeth ......
style hair ...... get dressed ...... other ......

Pain Management Strategies:

☐ deep breathing ☐ meditation
☐ visualization ☐ one object focus
☐ calming scents ☐ PMR
☐ rest ☐ music

Something that made me smile:
....
....

Something I am proud of: ....
....

Something I am grateful for: ....
....

Something I am looking forward to: ....
....

Lowest pain level today: 1 2 3 4 5
Highest pain level today: 1 2 3 4 5

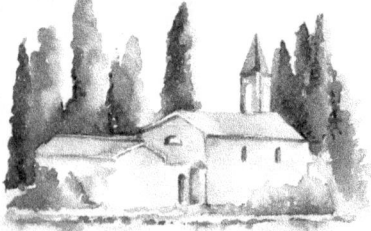

Sleep rating: 1 2 3 4 5

Mindset goal: ....
....

Eating goal: ....
....

Personal hygiene: bathe ......   teeth ......
style hair ......   get dressed ......   other ......

Pain Management Strategies:

- [ ] deep breathing
- [ ] visualization
- [ ] calming scents
- [ ] rest
- [ ] meditation
- [ ] one object focus
- [ ] PMR
- [ ] music

Something that made me smile:
....
....

Something I am proud of: ....
....

Something I am grateful for: ....
....

Something I am looking forward to: ....
....
....

Lowest pain level today: 1 2 3 4 5
Highest pain level today: 1 2 3 4 5

Friday........................

Sleep rating: 1 2 3 4 5

Mindset goal: ....
....

Eating goal: ....
....

Personal hygiene: bathe ......   teeth ......
style hair ......   get dressed ......   other ......

Pain Management Strategies:

- [ ] deep breathing
- [ ] visualization
- [ ] calming scents
- [ ] rest
- [ ] meditation
- [ ] one object focus
- [ ] PMR
- [ ] music

Something that made me smile:
....
....

Something I am proud of: ....
....

Something I am grateful for: ....
....

Something I am looking forward to: ....
....
....

Lowest pain level today: 1 2 3 4 5
Highest pain level today: 1 2 3 4 5

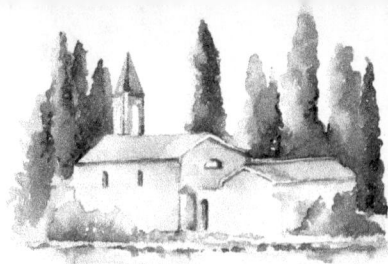

Week Twenty-Three

Saturday.....................

Sleep rating: 1 2 3 4 5

Mindset goal: ....
....

Eating goal: ....
....

Personal hygiene: bathe ......   teeth ......
style hair ......   get dressed ......   other ......

Pain Management Strategies:

☐ deep breathing   ☐ meditation
☐ visualization   ☐ one object focus
☐ calming scents   ☐ PMR
☐ rest   ☐ music

Something that made me smile:
....
....

Something I am proud of: ....
....

Something I am grateful for: ....
....

Something I am looking forward to: ....
....

Lowest pain level today: 1 2 3 4 5
Highest pain level today: 1 2 3 4 5

Sunday.........................

Sleep rating: 1 2 3 4 5

Mindset goal: ....
....

Eating goal: ....
....

Personal hygiene: bathe ......   teeth ......
style hair ......   get dressed ......   other ......

Pain Management Strategies:

☐ deep breathing   ☐ meditation
☐ visualization   ☐ one object focus
☐ calming scents   ☐ PMR
☐ rest   ☐ music

Something that made me smile:
....
....

Something I am proud of: ....
....

Something I am grateful for: ....
....

Something I am looking forward to: ....
....

Lowest pain level today: 1 2 3 4 5
Highest pain level today: 1 2 3 4 5

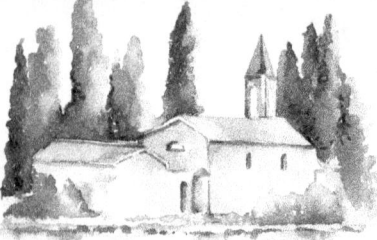

Week Twenty-Four

Goal for the week: ....
....

Days/Times I will leave the house or change settings: ....
....

When I will interact with friends or family: ....
....

Hobby I will work on: ....

Something new I'll try: ....

Medical tasks to do : ....
....
....

Monday.........................

Sleep rating: 1   2   3   4   5

Mindset goal: ....
....

Eating goal: ....
....

Personal hygiene: bathe ......   teeth ......
style hair ......   get dressed ......   other ......

Pain Management Strategies:

☐ deep breathing   ☐ meditation
☐ visualization   ☐ one object focus
☐ calming scents   ☐ PMR
☐ rest   ☐ music

Something that made me smile:
....
....
Something I am proud of: ....
....
Something I am grateful for: ....
....
Something I am looking forward to: ....
....
....
Lowest pain level today: 1 2 3 4 5
Highest pain level today: 1 2 3 4 5

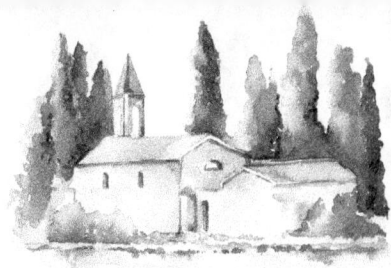

Sleep rating: 1 2 3 4 5

Mindset goal: ....

....

Eating goal: ....

....

Personal hygiene: bathe ......   teeth ......
style hair ......   get dressed ......   other ......

Pain Management Strategies:

☐ deep breathing ☐ meditation
☐ visualization   ☐ one object focus
☐ calming scents ☐ PMR
☐ rest   ☐ music

Something that made me smile:

....

....

Something I am proud of: ....

....

Something I am grateful for: ....

....

Something I am looking forward to: ....

....

....

Lowest pain level today: 1 2 3 4 5
Highest pain level today: 1 2 3 4 5

Wednesday.........................

Sleep rating: 1 2 3 4 5

Mindset goal: ....

....

Eating goal: ....

....

Personal hygiene: bathe ......   teeth ......
style hair ......   get dressed ......   other ......

Pain Management Strategies:

☐ deep breathing ☐ meditation
☐ visualization   ☐ one object focus
☐ calming scents ☐ PMR
☐ rest   ☐ music

Something that made me smile:

....

....

Something I am proud of: ....

....

Something I am grateful for: ....

....

....

Something I am looking forward to: ....

....

....

Lowest pain level today: 1 2 3 4 5
Highest pain level today: 1 2 3 4 5

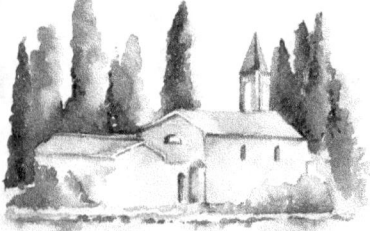

Thursday......................

Sleep rating: 1 2 3 4 5

Mindset goal: ....
....

Eating goal: ....
....

Personal hygiene: bathe ...... teeth ......
style hair ...... get dressed ...... other ......

Pain Management Strategies:

- [ ] deep breathing [ ] meditation
- [ ] visualization [ ] one object focus
- [ ] calming scents [ ] PMR
- [ ] rest [ ] music

Something that made me smile:
....
....

Something I am proud of: ....
....

Something I am grateful for: ....
....

Something I am looking forward to: ....
....
....

Lowest pain level today: 1 2 3 4 5
Highest pain level today: 1 2 3 4 5

Friday.........................

Sleep rating: 1 2 3 4 5

Mindset goal: ....
....

Eating goal: ....
....

Personal hygiene: bathe ...... teeth ......
style hair ...... get dressed ...... other ......

Pain Management Strategies:

- [ ] deep breathing [ ] meditation
- [ ] visualization [ ] one object focus
- [ ] calming scents [ ] PMR
- [ ] rest [ ] music

Something that made me smile:
....
....

Something I am proud of: ....
....

Something I am grateful for: ....
....

Something I am looking forward to: ....
....
....

Lowest pain level today: 1 2 3 4 5
Highest pain level today: 1 2 3 4 5

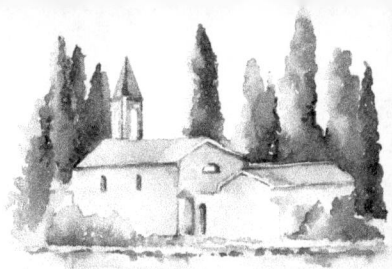

Week Twenty-Four

Saturday.....................

Sleep rating: 1 2 3 4 5

Mindset goal: ....
....

Eating goal: ....
....

Personal hygiene: bathe ......   teeth ......
style hair ......   get dressed ......   other ......

Pain Management Strategies:

☐ deep breathing   ☐ meditation
☐ visualization   ☐ one object focus
☐ calming scents   ☐ PMR
☐ rest   ☐ music

Something that made me smile:
....
....
Something I am proud of: ....
....
Something I am grateful for: ....
....
Something I am looking forward to: ....
....
....

Lowest pain level today: 1 2 3 4 5
Highest pain level today: 1 2 3 4 5

Sunday........................

Sleep rating: 1 2 3 4 5

Mindset goal: ....
....

Eating goal: ....
....

Personal hygiene: bathe ......   teeth ......
style hair ......   get dressed ......   other ......

Pain Management Strategies:

☐ deep breathing   ☐ meditation
☐ visualization   ☐ one object focus
☐ calming scents   ☐ PMR
☐ rest   ☐ music

Something that made me smile:
....
....
Something I am proud of: ....
....
Something I am grateful for: ....
....
....
Something I am looking forward to: ....
....
....

Lowest pain level today: 1 2 3 4 5
Highest pain level today: 1 2 3 4 5

Monthly Reflection

Think about how your mental health was this month. Did you use the strategies?
When were you your best? Your worst?

....

....

....

....

....

....

....

....

....

....

....

....

....

....

....

Happy Distraction

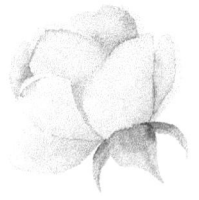

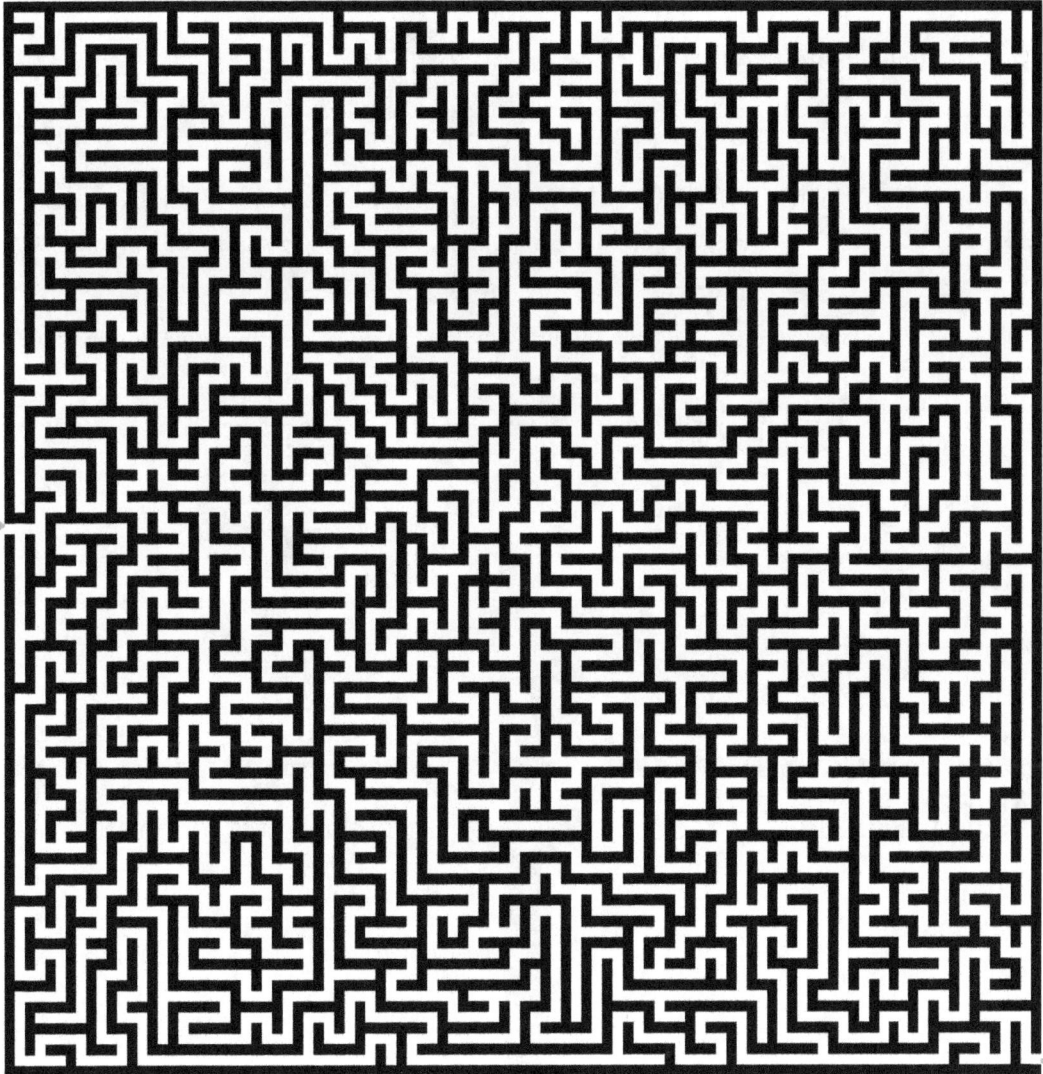

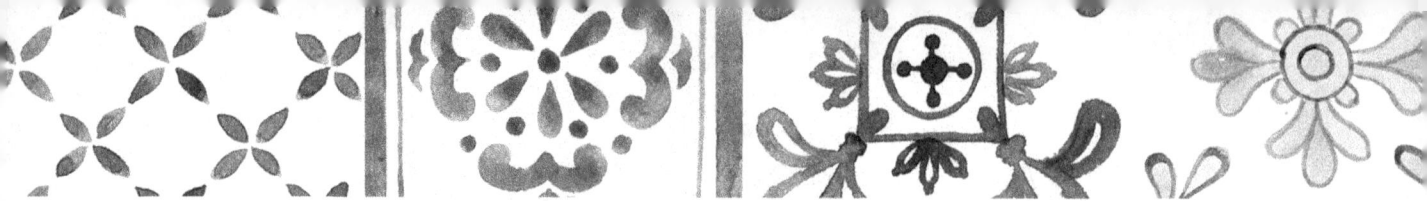

Week Twenty-Five

Goal for the week: ....
....

Days/Times I will leave the house or change settings: ....
....

When I will interact with friends or family: ....
....

Hobby I will work on: ....

Something new I'll try: ....

Medical tasks to do : ....
....
....

Monday.........................

Sleep rating: 1 2 3 4 5

Mindset goal: ....
....

Eating goal: ....
....

Personal hygiene: bathe ......   teeth ......
style hair ......   get dressed ......   other ......

Pain Management Strategies:

☐ deep breathing ☐ meditation
☐ visualization   ☐ one object focus
☐ calming scents ☐ PMR
☐ rest   ☐ music

Something that made me smile:
....
....
Something I am proud of: ....
....
Something I am grateful for: ....
....
....
Something I am looking forward to: ....
....
....
Lowest pain level today: 1 2 3 4 5
Highest pain level today: 1 2 3 4 5

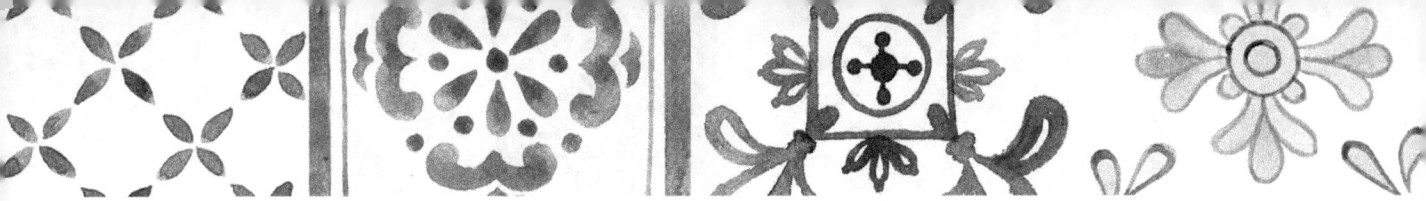

Tuesday..........................

Sleep rating: 1 2 3 4 5

Mindset goal: ....
....

Eating goal: ....
....

Personal hygiene: bathe ......   teeth ......
style hair ......   get dressed ......   other ......

Pain Management Strategies:

- ☐ deep breathing   ☐ meditation
- ☐ visualization   ☐ one object focus
- ☐ calming scents   ☐ PMR
- ☐ rest   ☐ music

Something that made me smile:
....
....
Something I am proud of: ....
....
Something I am grateful for: ....
....
Something I am looking forward to: ....
....
....
Lowest pain level today: 1 2 3 4 5
Highest pain level today: 1 2 3 4 5

Wednesday..........................

Sleep rating: 1 2 3 4 5

Mindset goal: ....
....

Eating goal: ....
....

Personal hygiene: bathe ......   teeth ......
style hair ......   get dressed ......   other ......

Pain Management Strategies:

- ☐ deep breathing   ☐ meditation
- ☐ visualization   ☐ one object focus
- ☐ calming scents   ☐ PMR
- ☐ rest   ☐ music

Something that made me smile:
....
....
Something I am proud of: ....
....
Something I am grateful for: ....
....
Something I am looking forward to: ....
....
....
Lowest pain level today: 1 2 3 4 5
Highest pain level today: 1 2 3 4 5

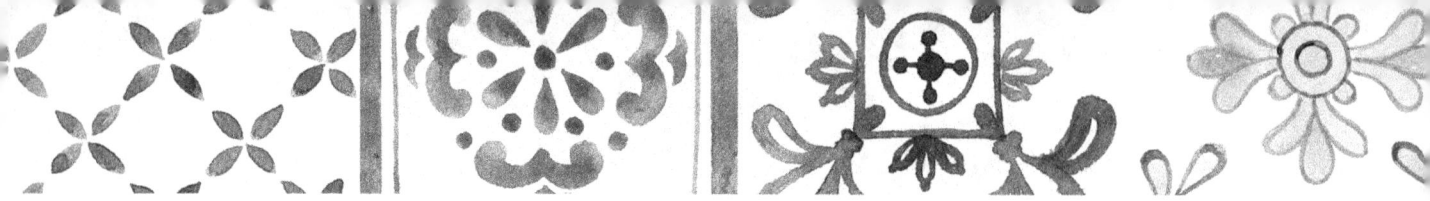

Thursday.....................

Sleep rating: 1 2 3 4 5

Mindset goal: ....
....

Eating goal: ....
....

Personal hygiene: bathe ......   teeth ......
style hair ......   get dressed ......   other ......

Pain Management Strategies:

- [ ] deep breathing [ ] meditation
- [ ] visualization [ ] one object focus
- [ ] calming scents [ ] PMR
- [ ] rest [ ] music

Something that made me smile:
....
....

Something I am proud of: ....
....

Something I am grateful for: ....
....

Something I am looking forward to: ....
....
....

Lowest pain level today: 1 2 3 4 5
Highest pain level today: 1 2 3 4 5

Friday..........................

Sleep rating: 1 2 3 4 5

Mindset goal: ....
....

Eating goal: ....
....

Personal hygiene: bathe ......   teeth ......
style hair ......   get dressed ......   other ......

Pain Management Strategies:

- [ ] deep breathing [ ] meditation
- [ ] visualization [ ] one object focus
- [ ] calming scents [ ] PMR
- [ ] rest [ ] music

Something that made me smile:
....
....

Something I am proud of: ....
....

Something I am grateful for: ....
....

Something I am looking forward to: ....
....
....

Lowest pain level today: 1 2 3 4 5
Highest pain level today: 1 2 3 4 5

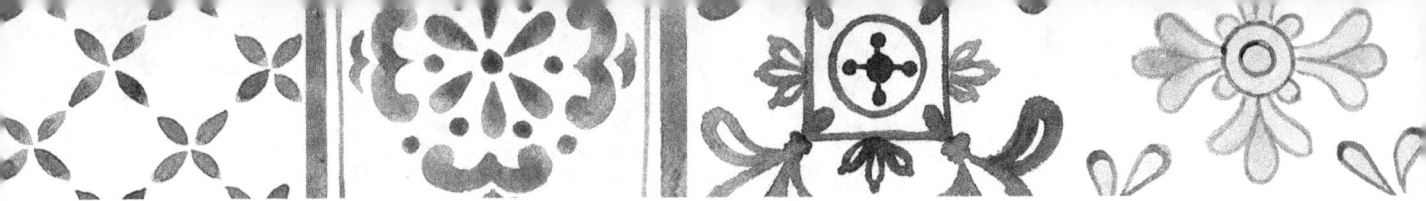

Saturday........................

Sleep rating: 1 2 3 4 5

Mindset goal: ....
....

Eating goal: ....
....

Personal hygiene: bathe ...... teeth ......
style hair ...... get dressed ...... other ......

Pain Management Strategies:

- [ ] deep breathing [ ] meditation
- [ ] visualization [ ] one object focus
- [ ] calming scents [ ] PMR
- [ ] rest [ ] music

Something that made me smile:
....
....
Something I am proud of: ....
....
Something I am grateful for: ....
....
Something I am looking forward to: ....
....

Lowest pain level today: 1 2 3 4 5
Highest pain level today: 1 2 3 4 5

Sunday........................

Sleep rating: 1 2 3 4 5

Mindset goal: ....
....

Eating goal: ....

Personal hygiene: bathe ...... teeth ......
style hair ...... get dressed ...... other ......

Pain Management Strategies:

- [ ] deep breathing [ ] meditation
- [ ] visualization [ ] one object focus
- [ ] calming scents [ ] PMR
- [ ] rest [ ] music

Something that made me smile:
....
....
Something I am proud of: ....
....
Something I am grateful for: ....
....
....
Something I am looking forward to: ....
....

Lowest pain level today: 1 2 3 4 5
Highest pain level today: 1 2 3 4 5

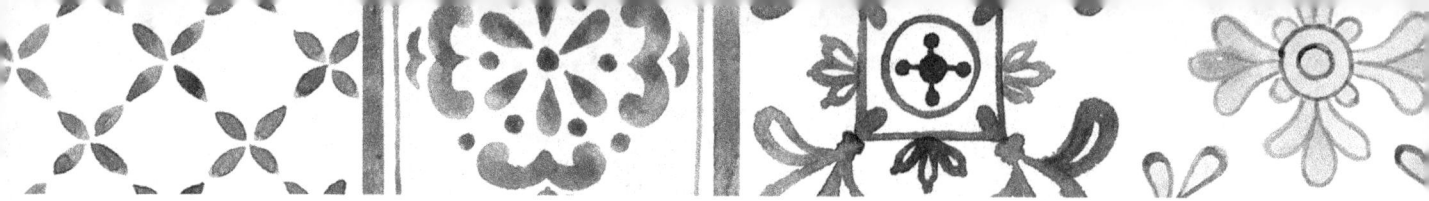

Week Twenty-Six

Goal for the week: ....
....

Days/Times I will leave the house or change settings: ....
....

When I will interact with friends or family: ....
....

Hobby I will work on: ....

Something new I'll try: ....

Medical tasks to do : ....
....
....

Monday.........................

Sleep rating: 1   2   3   4   5

Mindset goal: ....
....

Eating goal: ....
....

Personal hygiene: bathe ......   teeth ......
style hair ......   get dressed ......   other ......

Pain Management Strategies:

- [ ] deep breathing
- [ ] visualization
- [ ] calming scents
- [ ] rest
- [ ] meditation
- [ ] one object focus
- [ ] PMR
- [ ] music

Something that made me smile:
....
....

Something I am proud of: ....
....

Something I am grateful for: ....
....

Something I am looking forward to: ....
....
....

Lowest pain level today: 1 2 3 4 5
Highest pain level today: 1 2 3 4 5

Tuesday.......................

Sleep rating: 1 2 3 4 5

Mindset goal: ....
....

Eating goal: ....
....

Personal hygiene: bathe ...... teeth ......
style hair ...... get dressed ...... other ......

Pain Management Strategies:

☐ deep breathing ☐ meditation
☐ visualization ☐ one object focus
☐ calming scents ☐ PMR
☐ rest ☐ music

Something that made me smile:
....
....
Something I am proud of: ....
....
Something I am grateful for: ....
....
Something I am looking forward to: ....
....
....
Lowest pain level today: 1 2 3 4 5
Highest pain level today: 1 2 3 4 5

Wednesday...........................

Sleep rating: 1 2 3 4 5

Mindset goal: ....
....

Eating goal: ....
....

Personal hygiene: bathe ...... teeth ......
style hair ...... get dressed ...... other ......

Pain Management Strategies:

☐ deep breathing ☐ meditation
☐ visualization ☐ one object focus
☐ calming scents ☐ PMR
☐ rest ☐ music

Something that made me smile:
....
....
Something I am proud of: ....
....
Something I am grateful for: ....
....
....
Something I am looking forward to: ....
....
....
Lowest pain level today: 1 2 3 4 5
Highest pain level today: 1 2 3 4 5

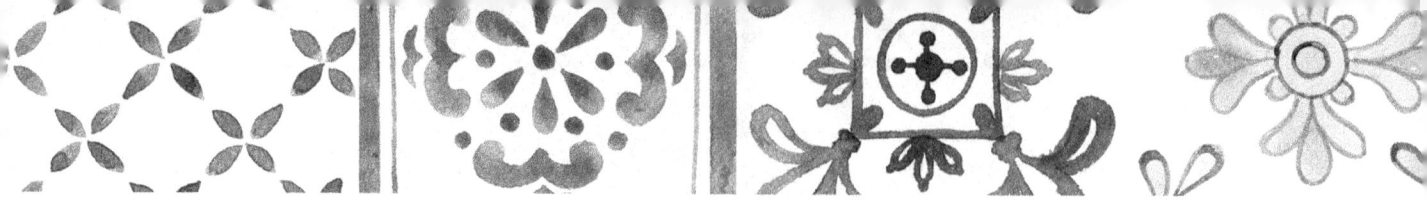

Thursday.....................

Sleep rating: 1 2 3 4 5

Mindset goal: ....
....

Eating goal: ....
....

Personal hygiene: bathe ...... teeth ......
style hair ...... get dressed ...... other ......

Pain Management Strategies:

- [ ] deep breathing [ ] meditation
- [ ] visualization [ ] one object focus
- [ ] calming scents [ ] PMR
- [ ] rest [ ] music

Something that made me smile:
....
....

Something I am proud of: ....
....

Something I am grateful for: ....
....

Something I am looking forward to: ....
....
....

Lowest pain level today: 1 2 3 4 5
Highest pain level today: 1 2 3 4 5

Friday........................

Sleep rating: 1 2 3 4 5

Mindset goal: ....
....

Eating goal: ....
....

Personal hygiene: bathe ...... teeth ......
style hair ...... get dressed ...... other ......

Pain Management Strategies:

- [ ] deep breathing [ ] meditation
- [ ] visualization [ ] one object focus
- [ ] calming scents [ ] PMR
- [ ] rest [ ] music

Something that made me smile:
....
....

Something I am proud of: ....
....

Something I am grateful for: ....
....

Something I am looking forward to: ....
....
....

Lowest pain level today: 1 2 3 4 5
Highest pain level today: 1 2 3 4 5

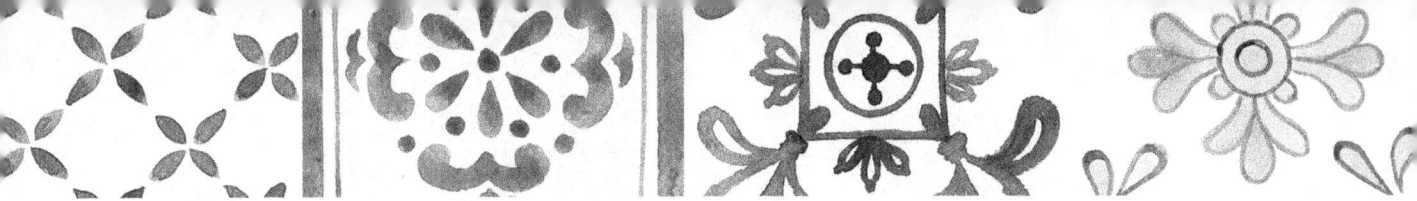

Saturday......................

Sleep rating: 1 2 3 4 5

Mindset goal: ....
....

Eating goal: ....
....

Personal hygiene: bathe ...... teeth ......
style hair ...... get dressed ...... other ......

Pain Management Strategies:

☐ deep breathing ☐ meditation
☐ visualization ☐ one object focus
☐ calming scents ☐ PMR
☐ rest ☐ music

Something that made me smile:
....
....
Something I am proud of: ....
....
Something I am grateful for: ....
....
Something I am looking forward to: ....
....
....
Lowest pain level today: 1 2 3 4 5
Highest pain level today: 1 2 3 4 5

Sunday.........................

Sleep rating: 1 2 3 4 5

Mindset goal: ....
....

Eating goal: ....
....

Personal hygiene: bathe ...... teeth ......
style hair ...... get dressed ...... other ......

Pain Management Strategies:

☐ deep breathing ☐ meditation
☐ visualization ☐ one object focus
☐ calming scents ☐ PMR
☐ rest ☐ music

Something that made me smile:
....
....
Something I am proud of: ....
....
Something I am grateful for: ....
....
Something I am looking forward to: ....
....
....
Lowest pain level today: 1 2 3 4 5
Highest pain level today: 1 2 3 4 5

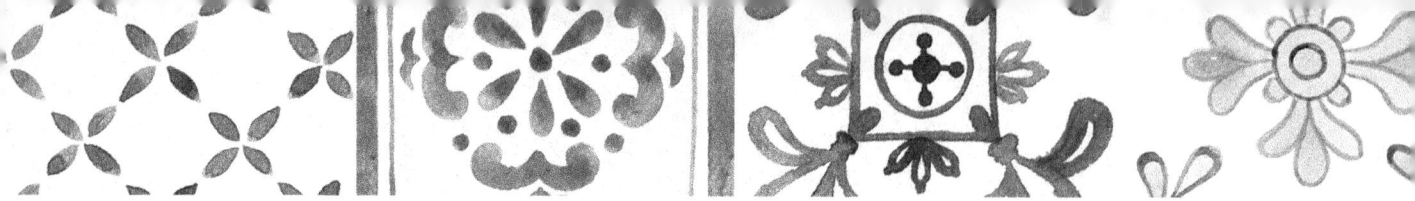

Week Twenty-Seven

Goal for the week: ....
....

Days/Times I will leave the house or change settings: ....
....

When I will interact with friends or family: ....
....

Hobby I will work on: ....

Something new I'll try: ....

Medical tasks to do : ....
....
....

Monday.......................

Sleep rating: 1   2   3   4   5

Mindset goal: ....
....

Eating goal: ....
....

Personal hygiene: bathe ......   teeth ......
style hair ......   get dressed ......   other ......

Pain Management Strategies:

- [ ] deep breathing
- [ ] visualization
- [ ] calming scents
- [ ] rest
- [ ] meditation
- [ ] one object focus
- [ ] PMR
- [ ] music

Something that made me smile:
....
....

Something I am proud of: ....
....

Something I am grateful for: ....
....

Something I am looking forward to: ....
....
....

Lowest pain level today: 1 2 3 4 5
Highest pain level today: 1 2 3 4 5

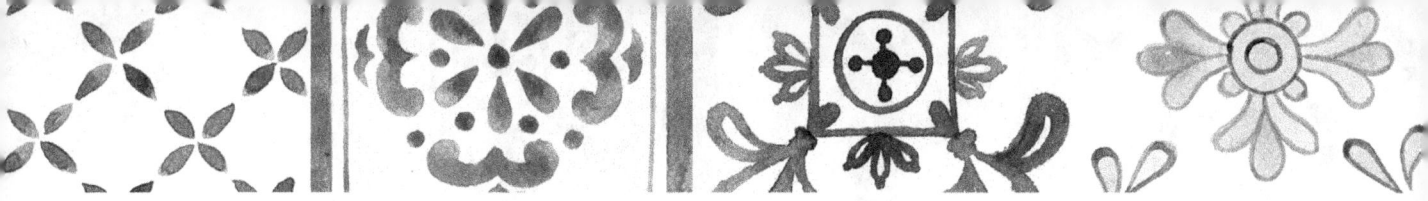

Tuesday....................... *Week Twenty-Seven*

Sleep rating: 1 2 3 4 5

Mindset goal: ....
....

Eating goal: ....
....

Personal hygiene: bathe ...... teeth ......
style hair ...... get dressed ...... other ......

Pain Management Strategies:

☐ deep breathing ☐ meditation
☐ visualization ☐ one object focus
☐ calming scents ☐ PMR
☐ rest ☐ music

Something that made me smile:
....
....

Something I am proud of: ....
....

Something I am grateful for: ....
....

Something I am looking forward to: ....
....
....

Lowest pain level today: 1 2 3 4 5
Highest pain level today: 1 2 3 4 5

Wednesday.........................

Sleep rating: 1 2 3 4 5

Mindset goal: ....
....

Eating goal: ....
....

Personal hygiene: bathe ...... teeth ......
style hair ...... get dressed ...... other ......

Pain Management Strategies:

☐ deep breathing ☐ meditation
☐ visualization ☐ one object focus
☐ calming scents ☐ PMR
☐ rest ☐ music

Something that made me smile:
....
....

Something I am proud of: ....
....

Something I am grateful for: ....
....

Something I am looking forward to: ....
....
....

Lowest pain level today: 1 2 3 4 5
Highest pain level today: 1 2 3 4 5

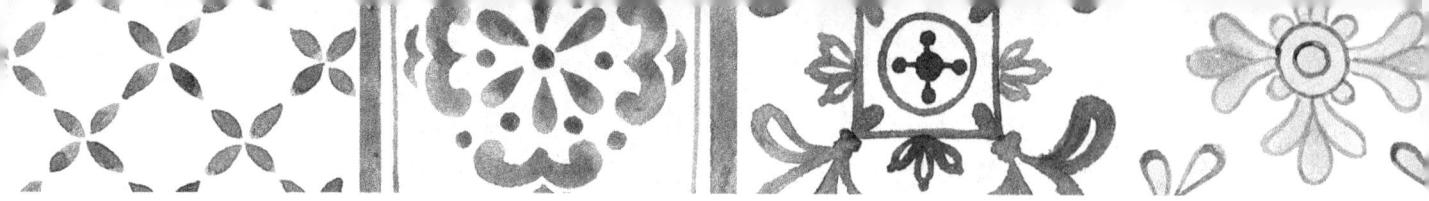

Sleep rating: 1 2 3 4 5

Mindset goal: ....
....

Eating goal: ....
....

Personal hygiene: bathe ...... teeth ......
style hair ...... get dressed ...... other ......

Pain Management Strategies:

☐ deep breathing ☐ meditation
☐ visualization ☐ one object focus
☐ calming scents ☐ PMR
☐ rest ☐ music

Something that made me smile:
....
....

Something I am proud of: ....
....

Something I am grateful for: ....
....

Something I am looking forward to: ....
....
....

Lowest pain level today: 1 2 3 4 5
Highest pain level today: 1 2 3 4 5

Friday..........................

Sleep rating: 1 2 3 4 5

Mindset goal: ....
....

Eating goal: ....
....

Personal hygiene: bathe ...... teeth ......
style hair ...... get dressed ...... other ......

Pain Management Strategies:

☐ deep breathing ☐ meditation
☐ visualization ☐ one object focus
☐ calming scents ☐ PMR
☐ rest ☐ music

Something that made me smile:
....
....

Something I am proud of: ....
....

Something I am grateful for: ....
....

Something I am looking forward to: ....
....
....

Lowest pain level today: 1 2 3 4 5
Highest pain level today: 1 2 3 4 5

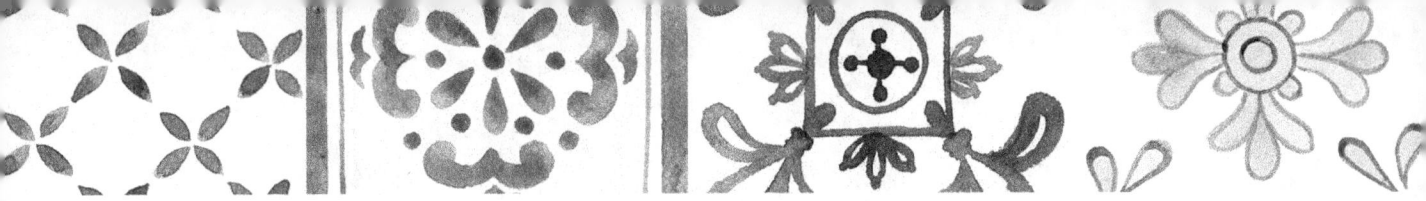

Saturday.......................

Sleep rating: 1 2 3 4 5

Mindset goal: ....
....

Eating goal: ....
....

Personal hygiene: bathe ...... teeth ......
style hair ...... get dressed ...... other ......

Pain Management Strategies:

☐ deep breathing ☐ meditation
☐ visualization ☐ one object focus
☐ calming scents ☐ PMR
☐ rest ☐ music

Something that made me smile:
....
....
Something I am proud of: ....
....
Something I am grateful for: ....
....
Something I am looking forward to: ....
....
....
Lowest pain level today: 1 2 3 4 5
Highest pain level today: 1 2 3 4 5

Sunday.........................

Sleep rating: 1 2 3 4 5

Mindset goal: ....
....

Eating goal: ....
....

Personal hygiene: bathe ...... teeth ......
style hair ...... get dressed ...... other ......

Pain Management Strategies:

☐ deep breathing ☐ meditation
☐ visualization ☐ one object focus
☐ calming scents ☐ PMR
☐ rest ☐ music

Something that made me smile:
....
....
Something I am proud of: ....
....
Something I am grateful for: ....
....
Something I am looking forward to: ....
....
....
Lowest pain level today: 1 2 3 4 5
Highest pain level today: 1 2 3 4 5

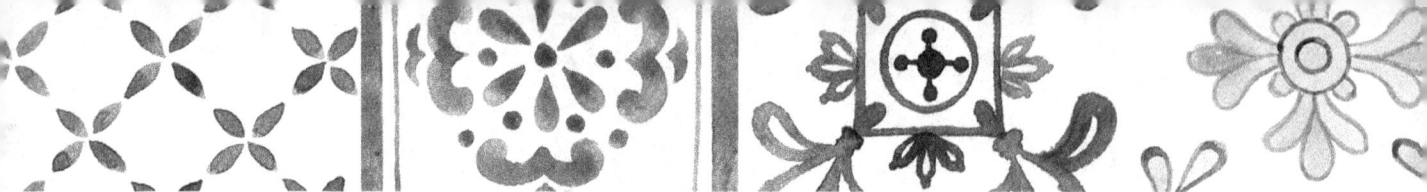

Week Twenty-Eight

Goal for the week: ....
....

Days/Times I will leave the house or change settings: ....
....

When I will interact with friends or family: ....
....

Hobby I will work on: ....

Something new I'll try: ....

Medical tasks to do : ....
....
....

Monday........................

Sleep rating: 1 2 3 4 5

Mindset goal: ....
....

Eating goal: ....
....

Personal hygiene: bathe ......   teeth ......
style hair ......   get dressed ......   other ......

Pain Management Strategies:

- ☐ deep breathing ☐ meditation
- ☐ visualization ☐ one object focus
- ☐ calming scents ☐ PMR
- ☐ rest ☐ music

Something that made me smile:
....
....
Something I am proud of: ....
....
Something I am grateful for: ....
....
Something I am looking forward to: ....
....
....
Lowest pain level today: 1 2 3 4 5
Highest pain level today: 1 2 3 4 5

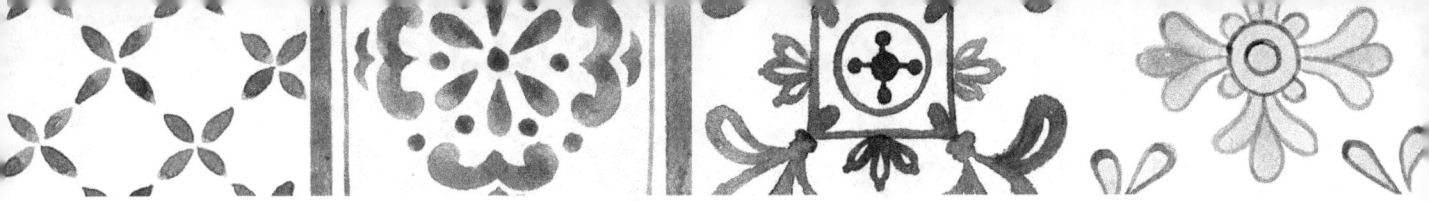

Week Twenty-Eight

Tuesday.........................

Sleep rating: 1 2 3 4 5

Mindset goal: ....
....

Eating goal: ....
....

Personal hygiene: bathe ......   teeth ......
style hair ......   get dressed ......   other ......

Pain Management Strategies:

- ☐ deep breathing
- ☐ visualization
- ☐ calming scents
- ☐ rest
- ☐ meditation
- ☐ one object focus
- ☐ PMR
- ☐ music

Something that made me smile:
....
....
Something I am proud of: ....
....
Something I am grateful for: ....
....
Something I am looking forward to: ....
....
....

Lowest pain level today: 1 2 3 4 5
Highest pain level today: 1 2 3 4 5

Wednesday.........................

Sleep rating: 1 2 3 4 5

Mindset goal: ....
....

Eating goal: ....
....

Personal hygiene: bathe ......   teeth ......
style hair ......   get dressed ......   other ......

Pain Management Strategies:

- ☐ deep breathing
- ☐ visualization
- ☐ calming scents
- ☐ rest
- ☐ meditation
- ☐ one object focus
- ☐ PMR
- ☐ music

Something that made me smile:
....
....
Something I am proud of: ....
....
Something I am grateful for: ....
....
Something I am looking forward to: ....
....
....

Lowest pain level today: 1 2 3 4 5
Highest pain level today: 1 2 3 4 5

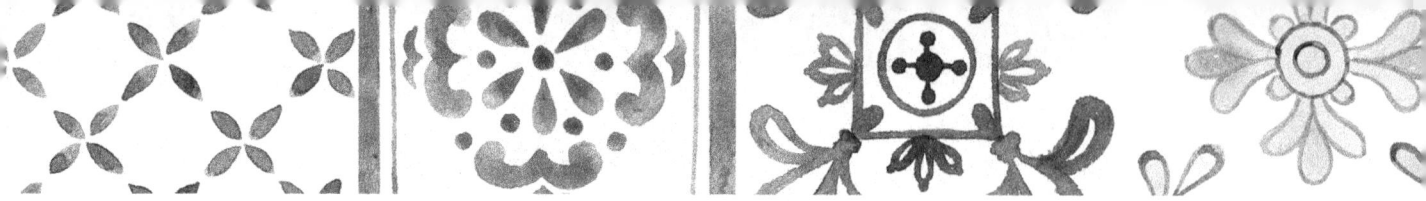

Sleep rating: 1 2 3 4 5

Mindset goal: ....
....

Eating goal: ....
....

Personal hygiene: bathe ......   teeth ......
style hair ......   get dressed ......   other ......

Pain Management Strategies:

☐ deep breathing ☐ meditation
☐ visualization ☐ one object focus
☐ calming scents ☐ PMR
☐ rest ☐ music

Something that made me smile:
....
....

Something I am proud of: ....
....

Something I am grateful for: ....
....

Something I am looking forward to: ....
....
....

Lowest pain level today: 1 2 3 4 5
Highest pain level today: 1 2 3 4 5

Friday.........................

Sleep rating: 1 2 3 4 5

Mindset goal: ....
....

Eating goal: ....
....

Personal hygiene: bathe ......   teeth ......
style hair ......   get dressed ......   other ......

Pain Management Strategies:

☐ deep breathing ☐ meditation
☐ visualization ☐ one object focus
☐ calming scents ☐ PMR
☐ rest ☐ music

Something that made me smile:
....
....

Something I am proud of: ....
....

Something I am grateful for: ....
....

Something I am looking forward to: ....
....
....

Lowest pain level today: 1 2 3 4 5
Highest pain level today: 1 2 3 4 5

Saturday.......................

Sleep rating: 1 2 3 4 5

Mindset goal: ....
....

Eating goal: ....
....

Personal hygiene: bathe ......   teeth ......
style hair ......   get dressed ......   other ......

Pain Management Strategies:

☐ deep breathing   ☐ meditation
☐ visualization   ☐ one object focus
☐ calming scents   ☐ PMR
☐ rest   ☐ music

Something that made me smile:
....
....
Something I am proud of: ....
....
Something I am grateful for: ....
....
Something I am looking forward to: ....
....
....
Lowest pain level today: 1 2 3 4 5
Highest pain level today: 1 2 3 4 5

Sunday.........................

Sleep rating: 1 2 3 4 5

Mindset goal: ....
....

Eating goal: ....
....

Personal hygiene: bathe ......   teeth ......
style hair ......   get dressed ......   other ......

Pain Management Strategies:

☐ deep breathing   ☐ meditation
☐ visualization   ☐ one object focus
☐ calming scents   ☐ PMR
☐ rest   ☐ music

Something that made me smile:
....
....
Something I am proud of: ....
....
Something I am grateful for: ....
....
....
Something I am looking forward to: ....
....
....
Lowest pain level today: 1 2 3 4 5
Highest pain level today: 1 2 3 4 5

Monthly Reflection

Think about how your mental health was this month. Did you use the strategies? When were you your best? Your worst?

....

....

....

....

....

....

....

....

....

....

....

....

....

....

....

....

....

....

Happy Distraction

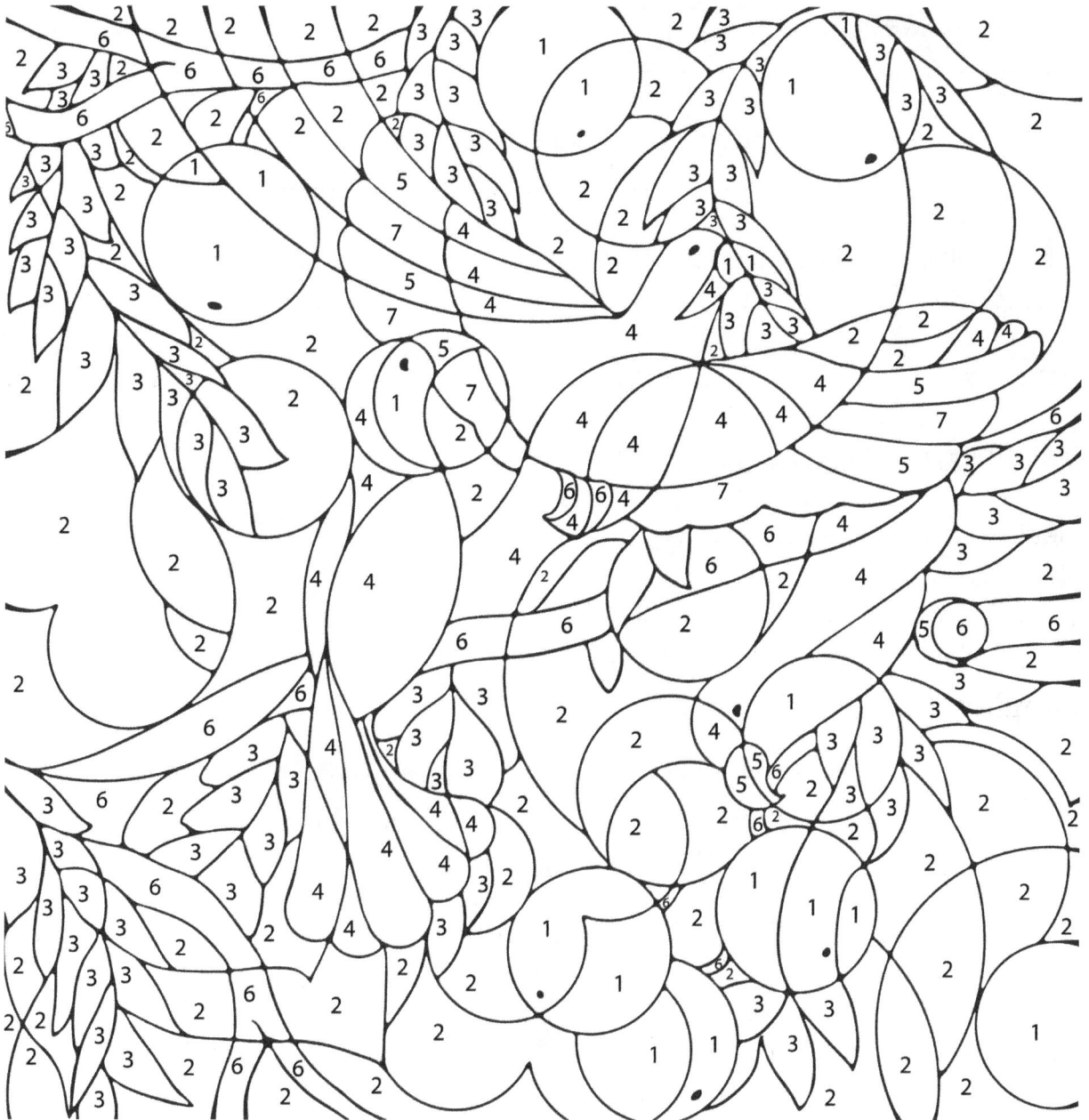

1 = orange   2 = dark green   3 = light green   4 = yellow   5 = gray

6 = brown   7 = light blue

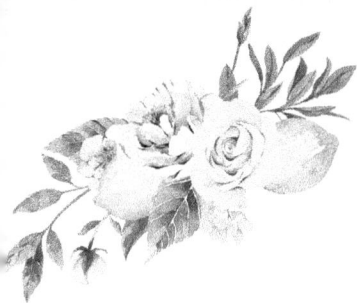

Week Twenty-Nine

Goal for the week: ....
....

Days/Times I will leave the house or change settings: ....
....

When I will interact with friends or family: ....
....

Hobby I will work on: ....

Something new I'll try: ....

Medical tasks to do : ....
....
....

Monday.........................

Sleep rating: 1 2 3 4 5

Mindset goal: ....
....

Eating goal: ....
....

Personal hygiene: bathe ...... teeth ......
style hair ...... get dressed ...... other ......

Pain Management Strategies:

☐ deep breathing ☐ meditation
☐ visualization ☐ one object focus
☐ calming scents ☐ PMR
☐ rest ☐ music

Something that made me smile:
....
....

Something I am proud of: ....
....

Something I am grateful for: ....
....

Something I am looking forward to: ....
....
....

Lowest pain level today: 1 2 3 4 5
Highest pain level today: 1 2 3 4 5

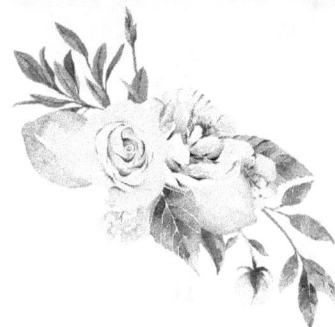

Week Twenty-Nine

Tuesday..........................

Sleep rating: 1 2 3 4 5

Mindset goal: ....
....

Eating goal: ....
....

Personal hygiene: bathe ......   teeth ......
style hair ......   get dressed ......   other ......

Pain Management Strategies:

- ☐ deep breathing
- ☐ visualization
- ☐ calming scents
- ☐ rest
- ☐ meditation
- ☐ one object focus
- ☐ PMR
- ☐ music

Something that made me smile:
....
....
Something I am proud of: ....
....
Something I am grateful for: ....
....
Something I am looking forward to: ....
....
....

Lowest pain level today: 1 2 3 4 5
Highest pain level today: 1 2 3 4 5

Wednesday.........................

Sleep rating: 1 2 3 4 5

Mindset goal: ....
....

Eating goal: ....
....

Personal hygiene: bathe ......   teeth ......
style hair ......   get dressed ......   other ......

Pain Management Strategies:

- ☐ deep breathing
- ☐ visualization
- ☐ calming scents
- ☐ rest
- ☐ meditation
- ☐ one object focus
- ☐ PMR
- ☐ music

Something that made me smile:
....
....
Something I am proud of: ....
....
Something I am grateful for: ....
....
Something I am looking forward to: ....
....
....

Lowest pain level today: 1 2 3 4 5
Highest pain level today: 1 2 3 4 5

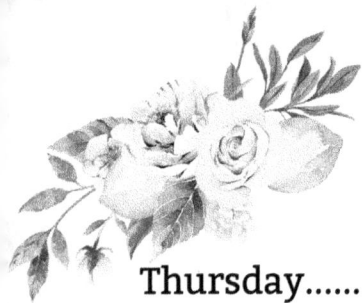

Thursday........................ *Week Twenty-Nine*

Sleep rating: 1 2 3 4 5

Mindset goal: ....
....

Eating goal: ....
....

Personal hygiene: bathe ...... teeth ......
style hair ...... get dressed ...... other ......

Pain Management Strategies:

☐ deep breathing ☐ meditation
☐ visualization ☐ one object focus
☐ calming scents ☐ PMR
☐ rest ☐ music

Something that made me smile:
....
....
Something I am proud of: ....
....
Something I am grateful for: ....
....
Something I am looking forward to: ....
....
....
Lowest pain level today: 1 2 3 4 5
Highest pain level today: 1 2 3 4 5

Friday..........................

Sleep rating: 1 2 3 4 5

Mindset goal: ....
....

Eating goal: ....
....

Personal hygiene: bathe ...... teeth ......
style hair ...... get dressed ...... other ......

Pain Management Strategies:

☐ deep breathing ☐ meditation
☐ visualization ☐ one object focus
☐ calming scents ☐ PMR
☐ rest ☐ music

Something that made me smile:
....
....
Something I am proud of: ....
....
Something I am grateful for: ....
....
Something I am looking forward to: ....
....
....
Lowest pain level today: 1 2 3 4 5
Highest pain level today: 1 2 3 4 5

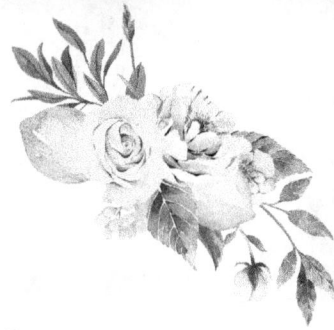

Saturday.....................

Week Twenty-Nine

Sleep rating: 1 2 3 4 5

Mindset goal: ....
....

Eating goal: ....
....

Personal hygiene: bathe ...... teeth ......
style hair ...... get dressed ...... other ......

Pain Management Strategies:

☐ deep breathing ☐ meditation
☐ visualization ☐ one object focus
☐ calming scents ☐ PMR
☐ rest ☐ music

Something that made me smile:
....
....

Something I am proud of: ....
....

Something I am grateful for: ....
....

Something I am looking forward to: ....
....

Lowest pain level today: 1 2 3 4 5
Highest pain level today: 1 2 3 4 5

Sunday........................

Sleep rating: 1 2 3 4 5

Mindset goal: ....
....

Eating goal: ....
....

Personal hygiene: bathe ...... teeth ......
style hair ...... get dressed ...... other ......

Pain Management Strategies:

☐ deep breathing ☐ meditation
☐ visualization ☐ one object focus
☐ calming scents ☐ PMR
☐ rest ☐ music

Something that made me smile:
....
....

Something I am proud of: ....
....

Something I am grateful for: ....
....

Something I am looking forward to: ....
....

Lowest pain level today: 1 2 3 4 5
Highest pain level today: 1 2 3 4 5

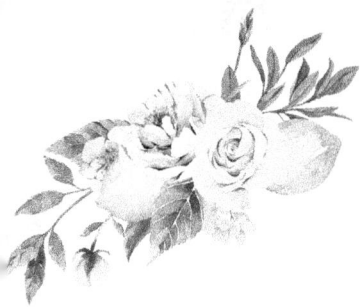

Week Thirty

Goal for the week: ....
....

Days/Times I will leave the house or change settings: ....
....

When I will interact with friends or family: ....
....

Hobby I will work on: ....

Something new I'll try: ....

Medical tasks to do : ....
....
....

Monday.........................

Sleep rating: 1 2 3 4 5

Mindset goal: ....
....

Eating goal: ....
....

Personal hygiene: bathe ...... teeth ......
style hair ...... get dressed ...... other ......

Pain Management Strategies:

☐ deep breathing ☐ meditation
☐ visualization   ☐ one object focus
☐ calming scents ☐ PMR
☐ rest   ☐ music

Something that made me smile:
....
....

Something I am proud of: ....
....

Something I am grateful for: ....
....
....

Something I am looking forward to: ....
....
....

Lowest pain level today: 1 2 3 4 5
Highest pain level today: 1 2 3 4 5

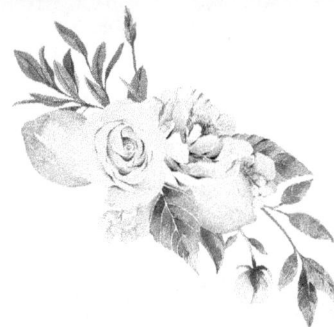

Week Thirty

Tuesday........................

Sleep rating: 1 2 3 4 5

Mindset goal: ....
....

Eating goal: ....
....

Personal hygiene: bathe ......   teeth ......
style hair ......   get dressed ......   other ......

Pain Management Strategies:

☐ deep breathing ☐ meditation
☐ visualization ☐ one object focus
☐ calming scents ☐ PMR
☐ rest ☐ music

Something that made me smile:
....
....
Something I am proud of: ....
....
Something I am grateful for: ....
....
Something I am looking forward to: ....
....
....
Lowest pain level today: 1 2 3 4 5
Highest pain level today: 1 2 3 4 5

Wednesday........................

Sleep rating: 1 2 3 4 5

Mindset goal: ....
....

Eating goal: ....
....

Personal hygiene: bathe ......   teeth ......
style hair ......   get dressed ......   other ......

Pain Management Strategies:

☐ deep breathing ☐ meditation
☐ visualization ☐ one object focus
☐ calming scents ☐ PMR
☐ rest ☐ music

Something that made me smile:
....
....
Something I am proud of: ....
....
Something I am grateful for: ....
....
Something I am looking forward to: ....
....
....
Lowest pain level today: 1 2 3 4 5
Highest pain level today: 1 2 3 4 5

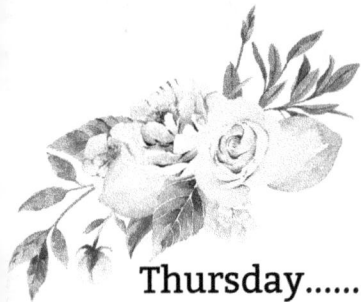

Thursday...................... *Week Thirty*

Sleep rating: 1 2 3 4 5

Mindset goal: ....

....

Eating goal: ....

....

Personal hygiene: bathe ...... teeth ......
style hair ...... get dressed ...... other ......

Pain Management Strategies:

☐ deep breathing ☐ meditation
☐ visualization ☐ one object focus
☐ calming scents ☐ PMR
☐ rest ☐ music

Something that made me smile:

....

....

Something I am proud of: ....

....

Something I am grateful for: ....

....

Something I am looking forward to: ....

....

....

Lowest pain level today: 1 2 3 4 5
Highest pain level today: 1 2 3 4 5

Friday.........................

Sleep rating: 1 2 3 4 5

Mindset goal: ....

....

Eating goal: ....

....

Personal hygiene: bathe ...... teeth ......
style hair ...... get dressed ...... other ......

Pain Management Strategies:

☐ deep breathing ☐ meditation
☐ visualization ☐ one object focus
☐ calming scents ☐ PMR
☐ rest ☐ music

Something that made me smile:

....

....

Something I am proud of: ....

....

Something I am grateful for: ....

....

Something I am looking forward to: ....

....

....

Lowest pain level today: 1 2 3 4 5
Highest pain level today: 1 2 3 4 5

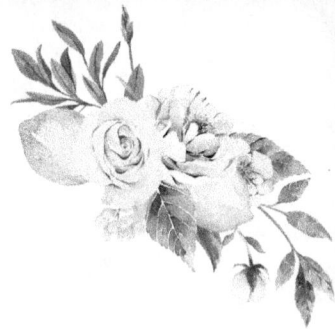

Week Thirty

Saturday.....................

Sleep rating: 1 2 3 4 5

Mindset goal: ....
....

Eating goal: ....
....

Personal hygiene: bathe ......   teeth ......
style hair ......   get dressed ......   other ......

Pain Management Strategies:

☐ deep breathing ☐ meditation
☐ visualization ☐ one object focus
☐ calming scents ☐ PMR
☐ rest ☐ music

Something that made me smile:
....
....

Something I am proud of: ....
....

Something I am grateful for: ....
....

Something I am looking forward to: ....
....

Lowest pain level today: 1 2 3 4 5
Highest pain level today: 1 2 3 4 5

Sunday........................

Sleep rating: 1 2 3 4 5

Mindset goal: ....
....

Eating goal: ....
....

Personal hygiene: bathe ......   teeth ......
style hair ......   get dressed ......   other ......

Pain Management Strategies:

☐ deep breathing ☐ meditation
☐ visualization ☐ one object focus
☐ calming scents ☐ PMR
☐ rest ☐ music

Something that made me smile:
....
....

Something I am proud of: ....
....

Something I am grateful for: ....
....

Something I am looking forward to: ....
....

Lowest pain level today: 1 2 3 4 5
Highest pain level today: 1 2 3 4 5

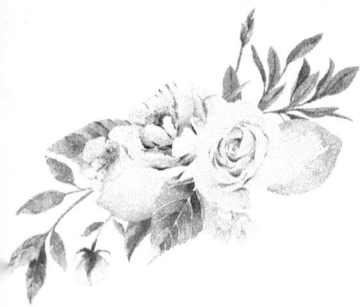

Week Thirty-One

Goal for the week: ....
....

Days/Times I will leave the house or change settings: ....
....

When I will interact with friends or family: ....
....

Hobby I will work on: ....

Something new I'll try: ....

Medical tasks to do : ....
....
....

Monday.........................

Sleep rating: 1 2 3 4 5

Mindset goal: ....
....

Eating goal: ....
....

Personal hygiene: bathe ......   teeth ......
style hair ......   get dressed ......   other ......

Pain Management Strategies:

- [ ] deep breathing
- [ ] visualization
- [ ] calming scents
- [ ] rest
- [ ] meditation
- [ ] one object focus
- [ ] PMR
- [ ] music

Something that made me smile:
....
....

Something I am proud of: ....
....

Something I am grateful for: ....
....
....

Something I am looking forward to: ....
....
....

Lowest pain level today: 1 2 3 4 5
Highest pain level today: 1 2 3 4 5

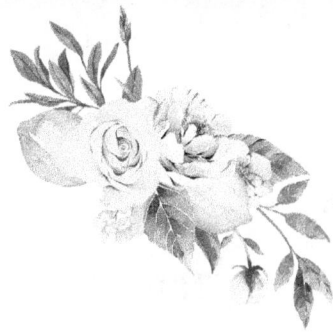

Sleep rating: 1 2 3 4 5

Mindset goal: ....

....

Eating goal: ....

....

Personal hygiene: bathe ...... teeth ......
style hair ...... get dressed ...... other ......

Pain Management Strategies:

☐ deep breathing ☐ meditation
☐ visualization ☐ one object focus
☐ calming scents ☐ PMR
☐ rest ☐ music

Something that made me smile:
....
....
Something I am proud of: ....
....
Something I am grateful for: ....
....
Something I am looking forward to: ....
....
....
Lowest pain level today: 1 2 3 4 5
Highest pain level today: 1 2 3 4 5

Wednesday.........................

Sleep rating: 1 2 3 4 5

Mindset goal: ....

....

Eating goal: ....

....

Personal hygiene: bathe ...... teeth ......
style hair ...... get dressed ...... other ......

Pain Management Strategies:

☐ deep breathing ☐ meditation
☐ visualization ☐ one object focus
☐ calming scents ☐ PMR
☐ rest ☐ music

Something that made me smile:
....
....
Something I am proud of: ....
....
Something I am grateful for: ....
....
Something I am looking forward to: ....
....
....
Lowest pain level today: 1 2 3 4 5
Highest pain level today: 1 2 3 4 5

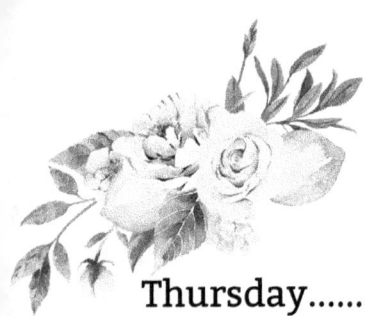

Thursday........................ *Week Thirty-One*

Sleep rating: 1 2 3 4 5

Mindset goal: ....
....

Eating goal: ....
....

Personal hygiene: bathe ......   teeth ......
style hair ......   get dressed ......   other ......

Pain Management Strategies:

- ☐ deep breathing
- ☐ visualization
- ☐ calming scents
- ☐ rest
- ☐ meditation
- ☐ one object focus
- ☐ PMR
- ☐ music

Something that made me smile:
....
....

Something I am proud of: ....
....

Something I am grateful for: ....
....

Something I am looking forward to: ....
....

Lowest pain level today: 1 2 3 4 5
Highest pain level today: 1 2 3 4 5

Friday...........................

Sleep rating: 1 2 3 4 5

Mindset goal: ....
....

Eating goal: ....
....

Personal hygiene: bathe ......   teeth ......
style hair ......   get dressed ......   other ......

Pain Management Strategies:

- ☐ deep breathing
- ☐ visualization
- ☐ calming scents
- ☐ rest
- ☐ meditation
- ☐ one object focus
- ☐ PMR
- ☐ music

Something that made me smile:
....
....

Something I am proud of: ....
....

Something I am grateful for: ....
....

Something I am looking forward to: ....
....

Lowest pain level today: 1 2 3 4 5
Highest pain level today: 1 2 3 4 5

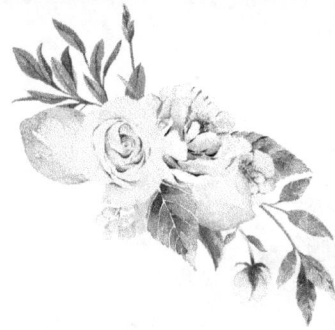

Week Thirty-One

Saturday......................

Sleep rating: 1 2 3 4 5

Mindset goal: ....
....

Eating goal: ....
....

Personal hygiene: bathe ......   teeth ......
style hair ......   get dressed ......   other ......

Pain Management Strategies:

- ☐ deep breathing ☐ meditation
- ☐ visualization ☐ one object focus
- ☐ calming scents ☐ PMR
- ☐ rest ☐ music

Something that made me smile:
....
....

Something I am proud of: ....
....

Something I am grateful for: ....
....

Something I am looking forward to: ....
....
....

Lowest pain level today: 1 2 3 4 5
Highest pain level today: 1 2 3 4 5

Sunday.........................

Sleep rating: 1 2 3 4 5

Mindset goal: ....
....

Eating goal: ....
....

Personal hygiene: bathe ......   teeth ......
style hair ......   get dressed ......   other ......

Pain Management Strategies:

- ☐ deep breathing ☐ meditation
- ☐ visualization ☐ one object focus
- ☐ calming scents ☐ PMR
- ☐ rest ☐ music

Something that made me smile:
....
....

Something I am proud of: ....
....

Something I am grateful for: ....
....

Something I am looking forward to: ....
....
....

Lowest pain level today: 1 2 3 4 5
Highest pain level today: 1 2 3 4 5

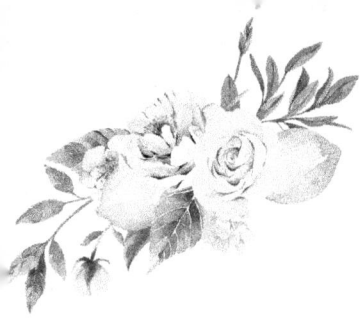

Week Thirty-Two

Goal for the week: ....
....

Days/Times I will leave the house or change settings: ....
....

When I will interact with friends or family: ....
....

Hobby I will work on: ....

Something new I'll try: ....

Medical tasks to do : ....
....
....

Monday...........................

Sleep rating: 1 2 3 4 5

Mindset goal: ....
....

Eating goal: ....
....

Personal hygiene: bathe ......   teeth ......
style hair ......   get dressed ......   other ......

Pain Management Strategies:

- ☐ deep breathing ☐ meditation
- ☐ visualization ☐ one object focus
- ☐ calming scents ☐ PMR
- ☐ rest ☐ music

Something that made me smile:
....
....

Something I am proud of: ....
....

Something I am grateful for: ....
....

Something I am looking forward to: ....
....
....

Lowest pain level today: 1 2 3 4 5
Highest pain level today: 1 2 3 4 5

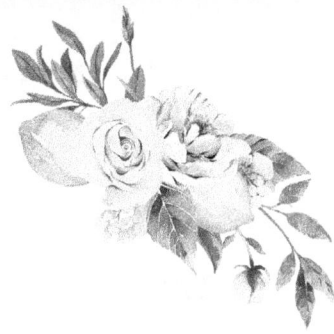

Week Thirty-Two

Tuesday...................

Sleep rating: 1 2 3 4 5

Mindset goal: ....
....

Eating goal: ....
....

Personal hygiene: bathe ...... teeth ......
style hair ...... get dressed ...... other ......

Pain Management Strategies:

☐ deep breathing ☐ meditation
☐ visualization ☐ one object focus
☐ calming scents ☐ PMR
☐ rest ☐ music

Something that made me smile:
....
....

Something I am proud of: ....
....

Something I am grateful for: ....
....

Something I am looking forward to: ....
....
....

Lowest pain level today: 1 2 3 4 5
Highest pain level today: 1 2 3 4 5

Wednesday.........................

Sleep rating: 1 2 3 4 5

Mindset goal: ....
....

Eating goal: ....
....

Personal hygiene: bathe ...... teeth ......
style hair ...... get dressed ...... other ......

Pain Management Strategies:

☐ deep breathing ☐ meditation
☐ visualization ☐ one object focus
☐ calming scents ☐ PMR
☐ rest ☐ music

Something that made me smile:
....
....

Something I am proud of: ....
....

Something I am grateful for: ....
....

Something I am looking forward to: ....
....
....

Lowest pain level today: 1 2 3 4 5
Highest pain level today: 1 2 3 4 5

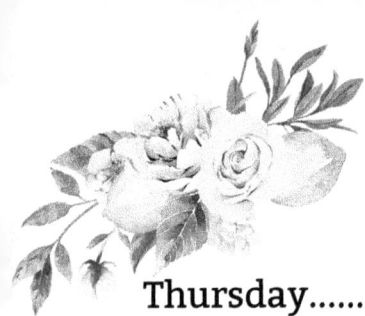

Sleep rating: 1 2 3 4 5

Mindset goal: ....
....

Eating goal: ....
....

Personal hygiene: bathe ...... teeth ......
style hair ...... get dressed ...... other ......

Pain Management Strategies:

- [ ] deep breathing
- [ ] visualization
- [ ] calming scents
- [ ] rest
- [ ] meditation
- [ ] one object focus
- [ ] PMR
- [ ] music

Something that made me smile:
....
....

Something I am proud of: ....
....

Something I am grateful for: ....
....

Something I am looking forward to: ....
....

Lowest pain level today: 1 2 3 4 5
Highest pain level today: 1 2 3 4 5

Friday.........................

Sleep rating: 1 2 3 4 5

Mindset goal: ....
....

Eating goal: ....
....

Personal hygiene: bathe ...... teeth ......
style hair ...... get dressed ...... other ......

Pain Management Strategies:

- [ ] deep breathing
- [ ] visualization
- [ ] calming scents
- [ ] rest
- [ ] meditation
- [ ] one object focus
- [ ] PMR
- [ ] music

Something that made me smile:
....
....

Something I am proud of: ....
....

Something I am grateful for: ....
....

Something I am looking forward to: ....
....

Lowest pain level today: 1 2 3 4 5
Highest pain level today: 1 2 3 4 5

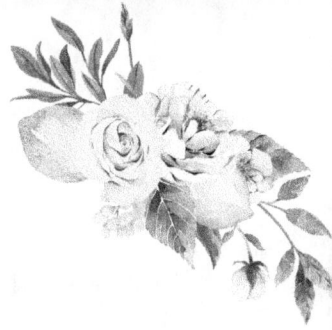

Saturday.................... *Week Thirty-Two*

Sleep rating: 1 2 3 4 5

Mindset goal: ....
....

Eating goal: ....
....

Personal hygiene: bathe ...... teeth ......
style hair ...... get dressed ...... other ......

Pain Management Strategies:

☐ deep breathing ☐ meditation
☐ visualization ☐ one object focus
☐ calming scents ☐ PMR
☐ rest ☐ music

Something that made me smile:
....
....

Something I am proud of: ....
....

Something I am grateful for: ....
....

Something I am looking forward to: ....
....

Lowest pain level today: 1 2 3 4 5
Highest pain level today: 1 2 3 4 5

Sunday........................

Sleep rating: 1 2 3 4 5

Mindset goal: ....
....

Eating goal: ....
....

Personal hygiene: bathe ...... teeth ......
style hair ...... get dressed ...... other ......

Pain Management Strategies:

☐ deep breathing ☐ meditation
☐ visualization ☐ one object focus
☐ calming scents ☐ PMR
☐ rest ☐ music

Something that made me smile:
....
....

Something I am proud of: ....
....

Something I am grateful for: ....
....

Something I am looking forward to: ....
....

Lowest pain level today: 1 2 3 4 5
Highest pain level today: 1 2 3 4 5

Monthly Reflection

Think about how your mental health was this month. Did you use the strategies?
When were you your best? Your worst?

....

....

....

....

....

....

....

....

....

....

....

....

....

....

....

....

....

....

Happy Distraction

Draw the other half of this plant. No pressure! Just have fun.

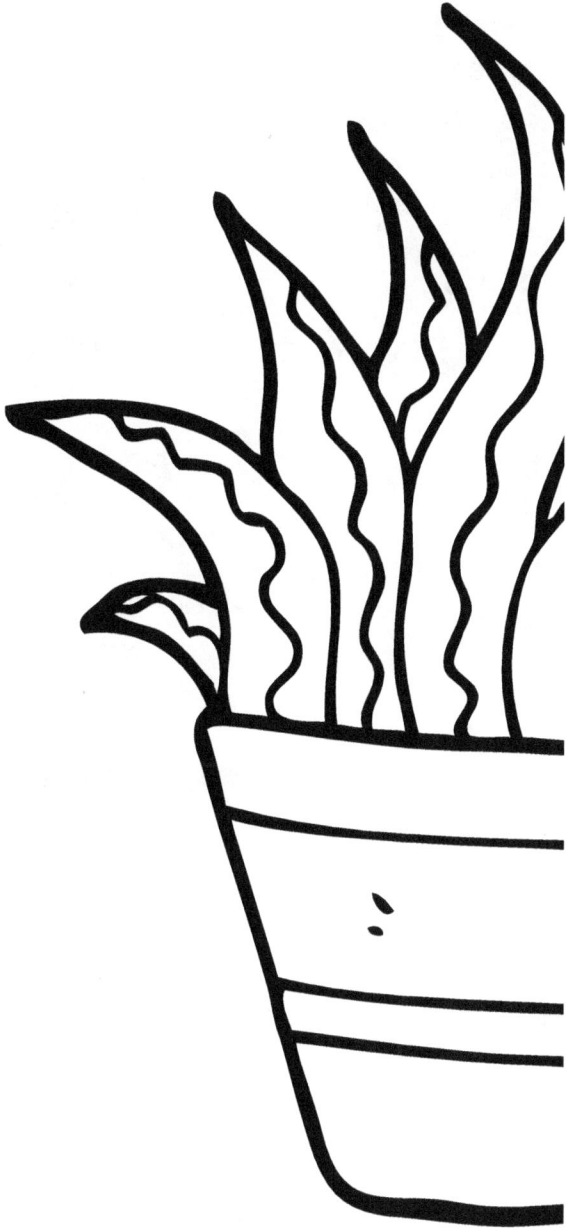

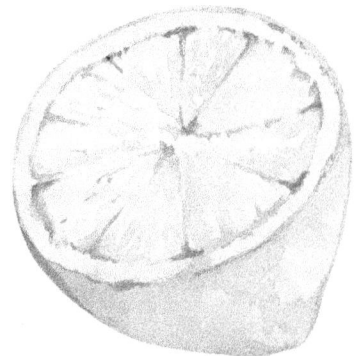

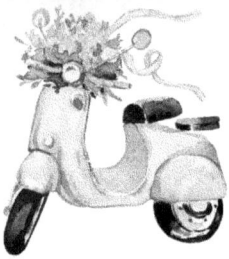

Week Thirty-Three

Goal for the week: ....
....

Days/Times I will leave the house or change settings: ....
....

When I will interact with friends or family: ....
....

Hobby I will work on: ....

Something new I'll try: ....

Medical tasks to do : ....
....
....

Monday.........................

Sleep rating: 1 2 3 4 5

Mindset goal: ....
....

Eating goal: ....
....

Personal hygiene: bathe ...... teeth ......
style hair ...... get dressed ...... other ......

Pain Management Strategies:

- [ ] deep breathing [ ] meditation
- [ ] visualization [ ] one object focus
- [ ] calming scents [ ] PMR
- [ ] rest [ ] music

Something that made me smile:
....
....

Something I am proud of: ....
....

Something I am grateful for: ....
....

Something I am looking forward to: ....
....

Lowest pain level today: 1 2 3 4 5
Highest pain level today: 1 2 3 4 5

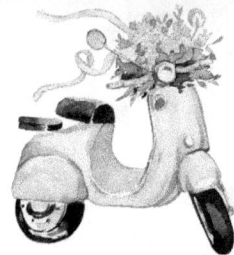

Tuesday.......................

Sleep rating: 1 2 3 4 5

Mindset goal: ....
....

Eating goal: ....
....

Personal hygiene: bathe ...... teeth ......
style hair ...... get dressed ...... other ......

Pain Management Strategies:

☐ deep breathing ☐ meditation
☐ visualization ☐ one object focus
☐ calming scents ☐ PMR
☐ rest ☐ music

Something that made me smile:
....
....
Something I am proud of: ....
....
Something I am grateful for: ....
....
Something I am looking forward to: ....
....
....

Lowest pain level today: 1 2 3 4 5
Highest pain level today: 1 2 3 4 5

Wednesday.........................

Sleep rating: 1 2 3 4 5

Mindset goal: ....
....

Eating goal: ....
....

Personal hygiene: bathe ...... teeth ......
style hair ...... get dressed ...... other ......

Pain Management Strategies:

☐ deep breathing ☐ meditation
☐ visualization ☐ one object focus
☐ calming scents ☐ PMR
☐ rest ☐ music

Something that made me smile:
....
....
Something I am proud of: ....
....
Something I am grateful for: ....
....
Something I am looking forward to: ....
....
....

Lowest pain level today: 1 2 3 4 5
Highest pain level today: 1 2 3 4 5

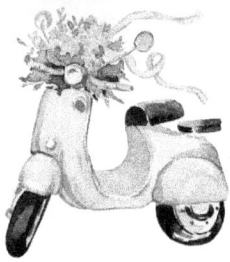

Thursday...................... *Week Thirty-Three*

Sleep rating: 1 2 3 4 5

Mindset goal: ....
....

Eating goal: ....
....

Personal hygiene: bathe ...... teeth ......
style hair ...... get dressed ...... other ......

Pain Management Strategies:

☐ deep breathing ☐ meditation
☐ visualization ☐ one object focus
☐ calming scents ☐ PMR
☐ rest ☐ music

Something that made me smile:
....
....

Something I am proud of: ....
....

Something I am grateful for: ....
....

Something I am looking forward to: ....
....
....

Lowest pain level today: 1 2 3 4 5
Highest pain level today: 1 2 3 4 5

Friday........................

Sleep rating: 1 2 3 4 5

Mindset goal: ....
....

Eating goal: ....
....

Personal hygiene: bathe ...... teeth ......
style hair ...... get dressed ...... other ......

Pain Management Strategies:

☐ deep breathing ☐ meditation
☐ visualization ☐ one object focus
☐ calming scents ☐ PMR
☐ rest ☐ music

Something that made me smile:
....
....

Something I am proud of: ....
....

Something I am grateful for: ....
....

Something I am looking forward to: ....
....
....

Lowest pain level today: 1 2 3 4 5
Highest pain level today: 1 2 3 4 5

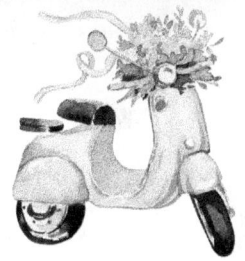

Week Thirty-Three

Saturday........................

Sleep rating: 1 2 3 4 5

Mindset goal: ....

....

Eating goal: ....

....

Personal hygiene: bathe ...... teeth ......
style hair ...... get dressed ...... other ......

Pain Management Strategies:

☐ deep breathing ☐ meditation
☐ visualization ☐ one object focus
☐ calming scents ☐ PMR
☐ rest ☐ music

Something that made me smile:

....

....

Something I am proud of: ....

....

Something I am grateful for: ....

....

Something I am looking forward to: ....

....

....

Lowest pain level today: 1 2 3 4 5
Highest pain level today: 1 2 3 4 5

Sunday..........................

Sleep rating: 1 2 3 4 5

Mindset goal: ....

....

Eating goal: ....

....

Personal hygiene: bathe ...... teeth ......
style hair ...... get dressed ...... other ......

Pain Management Strategies:

☐ deep breathing ☐ meditation
☐ visualization ☐ one object focus
☐ calming scents ☐ PMR
☐ rest ☐ music

Something that made me smile:

....

....

Something I am proud of: ....

....

Something I am grateful for: ....

....

Something I am looking forward to: ....

....

....

Lowest pain level today: 1 2 3 4 5
Highest pain level today: 1 2 3 4 5

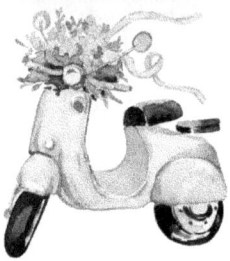

Week Thirty-Four

Goal for the week: ....
....

Days/Times I will leave the house or change settings: ....
....

When I will interact with friends or family: ....
....

Hobby I will work on: ....

Something new I'll try: ....

Medical tasks to do : ....
....
....

Monday.........................

Sleep rating: 1 2 3 4 5

Mindset goal: ....
....

Eating goal: ....
....

Personal hygiene: bathe ......   teeth ......
style hair ......   get dressed ......   other ......

Pain Management Strategies:

- [ ] deep breathing
- [ ] visualization
- [ ] calming scents
- [ ] rest
- [ ] meditation
- [ ] one object focus
- [ ] PMR
- [ ] music

Something that made me smile:
....
....
Something I am proud of: ....
....
Something I am grateful for: ....
....
Something I am looking forward to: ....
....
....
Lowest pain level today: 1 2 3 4 5
Highest pain level today: 1 2 3 4 5

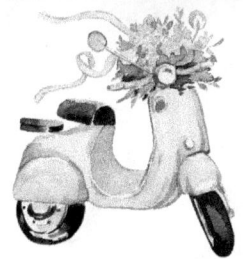

Sleep rating: 1 2 3 4 5

Mindset goal: ....
....

Eating goal: ....
....

Personal hygiene: bathe ......   teeth ......
style hair ......   get dressed ......   other ......

Pain Management Strategies:

☐ deep breathing ☐ meditation
☐ visualization ☐ one object focus
☐ calming scents ☐ PMR
☐ rest ☐ music

Something that made me smile:
....
....
Something I am proud of: ....
....
Something I am grateful for: ....
....
Something I am looking forward to: ....
....
....
Lowest pain level today: 1 2 3 4 5
Highest pain level today: 1 2 3 4 5

Wednesday..........................

Sleep rating: 1 2 3 4 5

Mindset goal: ....
....

Eating goal: ....
....

Personal hygiene: bathe ......   teeth ......
style hair ......   get dressed ......   other ......

Pain Management Strategies:

☐ deep breathing ☐ meditation
☐ visualization ☐ one object focus
☐ calming scents ☐ PMR
☐ rest ☐ music

Something that made me smile:
....
....
Something I am proud of: ....
....
Something I am grateful for: ....
....
Something I am looking forward to: ....
....
....
Lowest pain level today: 1 2 3 4 5
Highest pain level today: 1 2 3 4 5

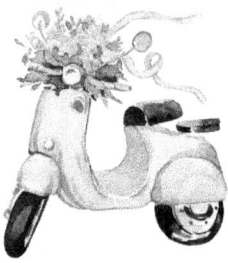

Thursday.....................

Week Thirty-Four

Sleep rating: 1 2 3 4 5

Mindset goal: ....
....

Eating goal: ....
....

Personal hygiene: bathe ......   teeth ......
style hair ......   get dressed ......   other ......

Pain Management Strategies:

- ☐ deep breathing ☐ meditation
- ☐ visualization ☐ one object focus
- ☐ calming scents ☐ PMR
- ☐ rest ☐ music

Something that made me smile:
....
....

Something I am proud of: ....
....

Something I am grateful for: ....
....

Something I am looking forward to: ....
....
....

Lowest pain level today: 1 2 3 4 5
Highest pain level today: 1 2 3 4 5

Friday.........................

Sleep rating: 1 2 3 4 5

Mindset goal: ....
....

Eating goal: ....
....

Personal hygiene: bathe ......   teeth ......
style hair ......   get dressed ......   other ......

Pain Management Strategies:

- ☐ deep breathing ☐ meditation
- ☐ visualization ☐ one object focus
- ☐ calming scents ☐ PMR
- ☐ rest ☐ music

Something that made me smile:
....
....

Something I am proud of: ....
....

Something I am grateful for: ....
....

Something I am looking forward to: ....
....
....

Lowest pain level today: 1 2 3 4 5
Highest pain level today: 1 2 3 4 5

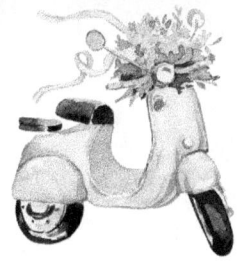

Sleep rating: 1 2 3 4 5

Mindset goal: ....

....

Eating goal: ....

....

Personal hygiene: bathe ......   teeth ......
style hair ......   get dressed ......   other ......

Pain Management Strategies:

☐ deep breathing   ☐ meditation
☐ visualization   ☐ one object focus
☐ calming scents   ☐ PMR
☐ rest   ☐ music

Something that made me smile:

....

....

Something I am proud of: ....

....

Something I am grateful for: ....

....

Something I am looking forward to: ....

....

....

Lowest pain level today: 1 2 3 4 5
Highest pain level today: 1 2 3 4 5

Sunday.........................

Sleep rating: 1 2 3 4 5

Mindset goal: ....

....

Eating goal: ....

....

Personal hygiene: bathe ......   teeth ......
style hair ......   get dressed ......   other ......

Pain Management Strategies:

☐ deep breathing   ☐ meditation
☐ visualization   ☐ one object focus
☐ calming scents   ☐ PMR
☐ rest   ☐ music

Something that made me smile:

....

....

Something I am proud of: ....

....

Something I am grateful for: ....

....

Something I am looking forward to: ....

....

....

Lowest pain level today: 1 2 3 4 5
Highest pain level today: 1 2 3 4 5

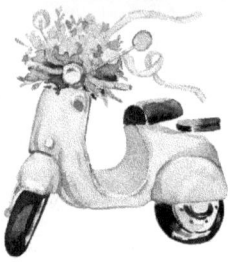

Week Thirty-Five

Goal for the week: ....
....

Days/Times I will leave the house or change settings: ....
....

When I will interact with friends or family: ....
....

Hobby I will work on: ....

Something new I'll try: ....

Medical tasks to do : ....
....
....

Monday.......................

Sleep rating: 1 2 3 4 5

Mindset goal: ....
....

Eating goal: ....
....

Personal hygiene: bathe ......   teeth ......
style hair ......   get dressed ......   other ......

Pain Management Strategies:

- [ ] deep breathing
- [ ] visualization
- [ ] calming scents
- [ ] rest
- [ ] meditation
- [ ] one object focus
- [ ] PMR
- [ ] music

Something that made me smile:
....
....
Something I am proud of: ....
....
Something I am grateful for: ....
....
Something I am looking forward to: ....
....
....
Lowest pain level today: 1 2 3 4 5
Highest pain level today: 1 2 3 4 5

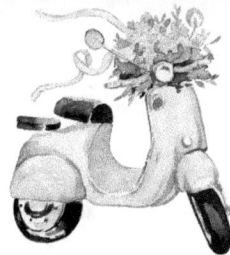

Week Thirty-Five

Tuesday............................

Sleep rating: 1 2 3 4 5

Mindset goal: ....
....

Eating goal: ....
....

Personal hygiene: bathe ......   teeth ......
style hair ......   get dressed ......   other ......

Pain Management Strategies:

- ☐ deep breathing
- ☐ visualization
- ☐ calming scents
- ☐ rest
- ☐ meditation
- ☐ one object focus
- ☐ PMR
- ☐ music

Something that made me smile:
....
....
Something I am proud of: ....
....
Something I am grateful for: ....
....
Something I am looking forward to: ....
....
....

Lowest pain level today: 1 2 3 4 5
Highest pain level today: 1 2 3 4 5

Wednesday............................

Sleep rating: 1 2 3 4 5

Mindset goal: ....
....

Eating goal: ....
....

Personal hygiene: bathe ......   teeth ......
style hair ......   get dressed ......   other ......

Pain Management Strategies:

- ☐ deep breathing
- ☐ visualization
- ☐ calming scents
- ☐ rest
- ☐ meditation
- ☐ one object focus
- ☐ PMR
- ☐ music

Something that made me smile:
....
....
Something I am proud of: ....
....
Something I am grateful for: ....
....
....
Something I am looking forward to: ....
....
....

Lowest pain level today: 1 2 3 4 5
Highest pain level today: 1 2 3 4 5

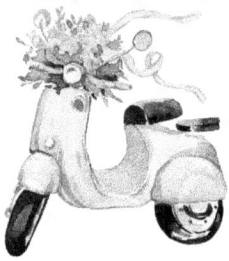

Thursday..................... Week Thirty-Five

Sleep rating: 1 2 3 4 5

Mindset goal: ....
....

Eating goal: ....
....

Personal hygiene: bathe ...... teeth ......
style hair ...... get dressed ...... other ......

Pain Management Strategies:

☐ deep breathing ☐ meditation
☐ visualization ☐ one object focus
☐ calming scents ☐ PMR
☐ rest ☐ music

Something that made me smile:
....
....

Something I am proud of: ....
....

Something I am grateful for: ....
....

Something I am looking forward to: ....
....
....

Lowest pain level today: 1 2 3 4 5
Highest pain level today: 1 2 3 4 5

Friday.........................

Sleep rating: 1 2 3 4 5

Mindset goal: ....
....

Eating goal: ....
....

Personal hygiene: bathe ...... teeth ......
style hair ...... get dressed ...... other ......

Pain Management Strategies:

☐ deep breathing ☐ meditation
☐ visualization ☐ one object focus
☐ calming scents ☐ PMR
☐ rest ☐ music

Something that made me smile:
....
....

Something I am proud of: ....
....

Something I am grateful for: ....
....

Something I am looking forward to: ....
....
....

Lowest pain level today: 1 2 3 4 5
Highest pain level today: 1 2 3 4 5

Saturday......................

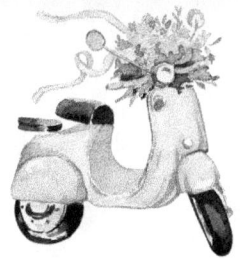

Week Thirty-Five

Sleep rating: 1 2 3 4 5

Mindset goal: ....
....

Eating goal: ....
....

Personal hygiene: bathe ......   teeth ......
style hair ......   get dressed ......   other ......

Pain Management Strategies:

- [ ] deep breathing [ ] meditation
- [ ] visualization [ ] one object focus
- [ ] calming scents [ ] PMR
- [ ] rest [ ] music

Something that made me smile:
....
....
Something I am proud of: ....
....
....
Something I am grateful for: ....
....
....
Something I am looking forward to: ....
....
....
Lowest pain level today: 1 2 3 4 5
Highest pain level today: 1 2 3 4 5

Sunday.......................

Sleep rating: 1 2 3 4 5

Mindset goal: ....
....

Eating goal: ....
....

Personal hygiene: bathe ......   teeth ......
style hair ......   get dressed ......   other ......

Pain Management Strategies:

- [ ] deep breathing [ ] meditation
- [ ] visualization [ ] one object focus
- [ ] calming scents [ ] PMR
- [ ] rest [ ] music

Something that made me smile:
....
....
Something I am proud of: ....
....
....
Something I am grateful for: ....
....
....
Something I am looking forward to: ....
....
....
Lowest pain level today: 1 2 3 4 5
Highest pain level today: 1 2 3 4 5

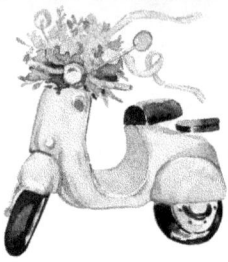

Week Thirty-Six

Goal for the week: ....
....

Days/Times I will leave the house or change settings: ....
....

When I will interact with friends or family: ....
....

Hobby I will work on: ....

Something new I'll try: ....

Medical tasks to do : ....
....
....

Monday........................

Sleep rating: 1   2   3   4   5

Mindset goal: ....
....

Eating goal: ....
....

Personal hygiene: bathe ......   teeth ......
style hair ......   get dressed ......   other ......

Pain Management Strategies:

☐ deep breathing ☐ meditation
☐ visualization   ☐ one object focus
☐ calming scents ☐ PMR
☐ rest   ☐ music

Something that made me smile:
....
....

Something I am proud of: ....
....

Something I am grateful for: ....
....

Something I am looking forward to: ....
....
....

Lowest pain level today: 1 2 3 4 5
Highest pain level today: 1 2 3 4 5

Tuesday.....................

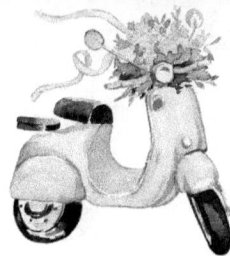

Week Thirty-Six

Sleep rating: 1 2 3 4 5

Mindset goal: ....
....

Eating goal: ....
....

Personal hygiene: bathe ...... teeth ......
style hair ...... get dressed ...... other ......

Pain Management Strategies:

☐ deep breathing ☐ meditation
☐ visualization ☐ one object focus
☐ calming scents ☐ PMR
☐ rest ☐ music

Something that made me smile:
....
....
Something I am proud of: ....
....
Something I am grateful for: ....
....
Something I am looking forward to: ....
....

Lowest pain level today: 1 2 3 4 5
Highest pain level today: 1 2 3 4 5

Wednesday..........................

Sleep rating: 1 2 3 4 5

Mindset goal: ....
....

Eating goal: ....
....

Personal hygiene: bathe ...... teeth ......
style hair ...... get dressed ...... other ......

Pain Management Strategies:

☐ deep breathing ☐ meditation
☐ visualization ☐ one object focus
☐ calming scents ☐ PMR
☐ rest ☐ music

Something that made me smile:
....
....
Something I am proud of: ....
....
Something I am grateful for: ....
....
Something I am looking forward to: ....
....

Lowest pain level today: 1 2 3 4 5
Highest pain level today: 1 2 3 4 5

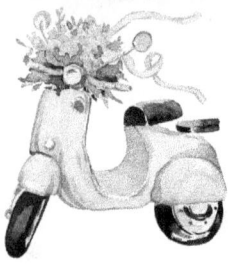

Thursday..................... *Week Thirty-Six*

Sleep rating: 1 2 3 4 5

Mindset goal: ....
....

Eating goal: ....
....

Personal hygiene: bathe ...... teeth ......
style hair ...... get dressed ...... other ......

Pain Management Strategies:

- [ ] deep breathing
- [ ] meditation
- [ ] visualization
- [ ] one object focus
- [ ] calming scents
- [ ] PMR
- [ ] rest
- [ ] music

Something that made me smile:
....
....

Something I am proud of: ....
....

Something I am grateful for: ....
....

Something I am looking forward to: ....
....

Lowest pain level today: 1 2 3 4 5
Highest pain level today: 1 2 3 4 5

Friday........................

Sleep rating: 1 2 3 4 5

Mindset goal: ....
....

Eating goal: ....
....

Personal hygiene: bathe ...... teeth ......
style hair ...... get dressed ...... other ......

Pain Management Strategies:

- [ ] deep breathing
- [ ] meditation
- [ ] visualization
- [ ] one object focus
- [ ] calming scents
- [ ] PMR
- [ ] rest
- [ ] music

Something that made me smile:
....
....

Something I am proud of: ....
....

Something I am grateful for: ....
....

Something I am looking forward to: ....
....

Lowest pain level today: 1 2 3 4 5
Highest pain level today: 1 2 3 4 5

Saturday......................

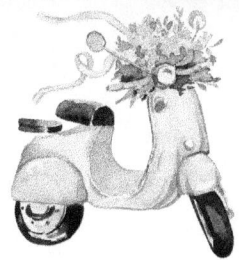

Week Thirty-Six

Sleep rating: 1 2 3 4 5

Mindset goal: ....
....

Eating goal: ....
....

Personal hygiene: bathe ......   teeth ......
style hair ......   get dressed ......   other ......

Pain Management Strategies:

☐ deep breathing ☐ meditation
☐ visualization ☐ one object focus
☐ calming scents ☐ PMR
☐ rest ☐ music

Something that made me smile:
....
....
Something I am proud of: ....
....
....
Something I am grateful for: ....
....
....
Something I am looking forward to: ....
....
....
Lowest pain level today: 1 2 3 4 5
Highest pain level today: 1 2 3 4 5

Sunday........................

Sleep rating: 1 2 3 4 5

Mindset goal: ....
....

Eating goal: ....
....

Personal hygiene: bathe ......   teeth ......
style hair ......   get dressed ......   other ......

Pain Management Strategies:

☐ deep breathing ☐ meditation
☐ visualization ☐ one object focus
☐ calming scents ☐ PMR
☐ rest ☐ music

Something that made me smile:
....
....
Something I am proud of: ....
....
....
Something I am grateful for: ....
....
....
Something I am looking forward to: ....
....
....
Lowest pain level today: 1 2 3 4 5
Highest pain level today: 1 2 3 4 5

Monthly Reflection

Think about how your mental health was this month. Did you use the strategies?
When were you your best? Your worst?

....

....

....

....

....

....

....

....

....

....

....

....

....

....

....

....

....

....

....

Happy Distraction

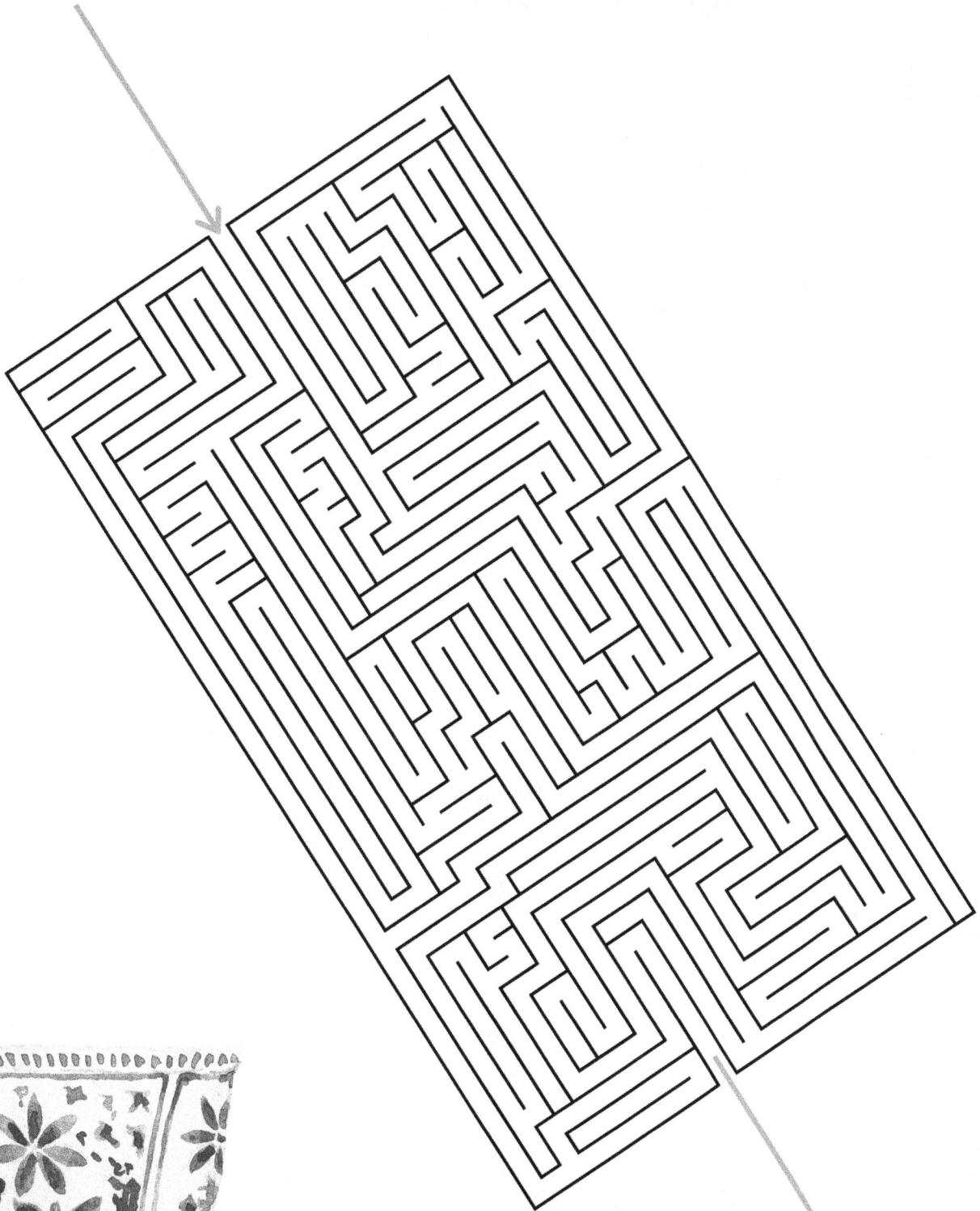

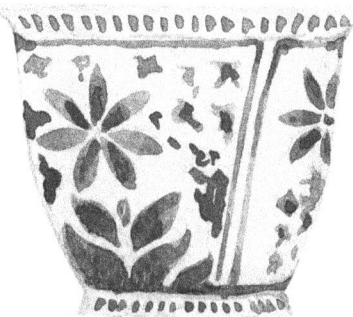

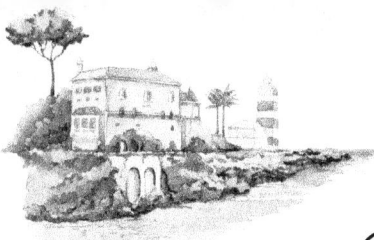

Week Thirty-Seven

Goal for the week: ....
....

Days/Times I will leave the house or change settings: ....
....

When I will interact with friends or family: ....
....

Hobby I will work on: ....

Something new I'll try: ....

Medical tasks to do : ....
....
....

Monday.........................

Sleep rating: 1 2 3 4 5

Mindset goal: ....
....

Eating goal: ....
....

Personal hygiene: bathe ......   teeth ......
style hair ......   get dressed ......   other ......

Pain Management Strategies:

☐ deep breathing ☐ meditation
☐ visualization   ☐ one object focus
☐ calming scents ☐ PMR
☐ rest   ☐ music

Something that made me smile:
....
....

Something I am proud of: ....
....

Something I am grateful for: ....
....

Something I am looking forward to: ....
....
....

Lowest pain level today: 1 2 3 4 5
Highest pain level today: 1 2 3 4 5

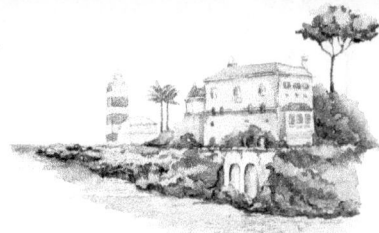

Tuesday.........................

Sleep rating: 1 2 3 4 5

Mindset goal: ....
....

Eating goal: ....
....

Personal hygiene: bathe ......   teeth ......
style hair ......   get dressed ......   other ......

Pain Management Strategies:

☐ deep breathing ☐ meditation
☐ visualization ☐ one object focus
☐ calming scents ☐ PMR
☐ rest ☐ music

Something that made me smile:
....
....
Something I am proud of: ....
....
Something I am grateful for: ....
....
Something I am looking forward to: ....
....
....
Lowest pain level today: 1 2 3 4 5
Highest pain level today: 1 2 3 4 5

Wednesday.........................

Sleep rating: 1 2 3 4 5

Mindset goal: ....
....

Eating goal: ....
....

Personal hygiene: bathe ......   teeth ......
style hair ......   get dressed ......   other ......

Pain Management Strategies:

☐ deep breathing ☐ meditation
☐ visualization ☐ one object focus
☐ calming scents ☐ PMR
☐ rest ☐ music

Something that made me smile:
....
....
Something I am proud of: ....
....
Something I am grateful for: ....
....
Something I am looking forward to: ....
....
....
Lowest pain level today: 1 2 3 4 5
Highest pain level today: 1 2 3 4 5

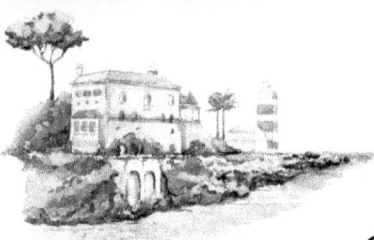

Sleep rating: 1 2 3 4 5

Mindset goal: ....
....

Eating goal: ....
....

Personal hygiene: bathe ...... teeth ......
style hair ...... get dressed ...... other ......

Pain Management Strategies:

☐ deep breathing ☐ meditation
☐ visualization ☐ one object focus
☐ calming scents ☐ PMR
☐ rest ☐ music

Something that made me smile:
....
....

Something I am proud of: ....
....

Something I am grateful for: ....
....

Something I am looking forward to: ....
....
....

Lowest pain level today: 1 2 3 4 5
Highest pain level today: 1 2 3 4 5

Friday.........................

Sleep rating: 1 2 3 4 5

Mindset goal: ....
....

Eating goal: ....
....

Personal hygiene: bathe ...... teeth ......
style hair ...... get dressed ...... other ......

Pain Management Strategies:

☐ deep breathing ☐ meditation
☐ visualization ☐ one object focus
☐ calming scents ☐ PMR
☐ rest ☐ music

Something that made me smile:
....
....

Something I am proud of: ....
....

Something I am grateful for: ....
....

Something I am looking forward to: ....
....
....

Lowest pain level today: 1 2 3 4 5
Highest pain level today: 1 2 3 4 5

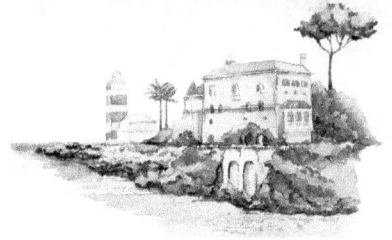

Saturday........................

Sleep rating: 1 2 3 4 5

Mindset goal: ....

....

Eating goal: ....

....

Personal hygiene: bathe ......   teeth ......
style hair ......   get dressed ......   other ......

Pain Management Strategies:

☐ deep breathing ☐ meditation
☐ visualization ☐ one object focus
☐ calming scents ☐ PMR
☐ rest ☐ music

Something that made me smile:

....

....

Something I am proud of: ....

....

Something I am grateful for: ....

....

Something I am looking forward to: ....

....

....

Lowest pain level today: 1 2 3 4 5
Highest pain level today: 1 2 3 4 5

Sunday........................

Sleep rating: 1 2 3 4 5

Mindset goal: ....

....

Eating goal: ....

....

Personal hygiene: bathe ......   teeth ......
style hair ......   get dressed ......   other ......

Pain Management Strategies:

☐ deep breathing ☐ meditation
☐ visualization ☐ one object focus
☐ calming scents ☐ PMR
☐ rest ☐ music

Something that made me smile:

....

....

Something I am proud of: ....

....

Something I am grateful for: ....

....

Something I am looking forward to: ....

....

....

Lowest pain level today: 1 2 3 4 5
Highest pain level today: 1 2 3 4 5

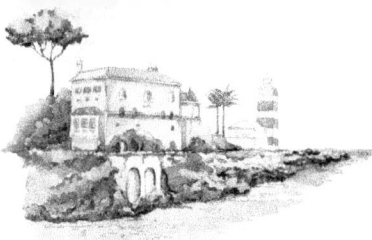

Week Thirty-Eight

Goal for the week: ....
....

Days/Times I will leave the house or change settings: ....
....

When I will interact with friends or family: ....
....

Hobby I will work on: ....

Something new I'll try: ....

Medical tasks to do : ....
....
....

Monday........................

Sleep rating: 1   2   3   4   5

Mindset goal: ....
....

Eating goal: ....
....

Personal hygiene: bathe ......   teeth ......
style hair ......   get dressed ......   other ......

Pain Management Strategies:

- [ ] deep breathing
- [ ] visualization
- [ ] calming scents
- [ ] rest
- [ ] meditation
- [ ] one object focus
- [ ] PMR
- [ ] music

Something that made me smile:
....
....

Something I am proud of: ....
....

Something I am grateful for: ....
....

Something I am looking forward to: ....
....
....

Lowest pain level today: 1 2 3 4 5
Highest pain level today: 1 2 3 4 5

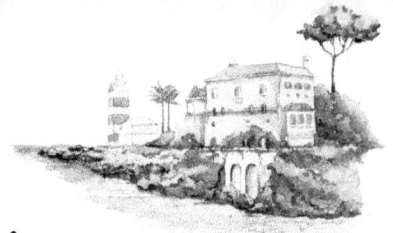

Sleep rating: 1 2 3 4 5

Mindset goal: ....
....

Eating goal: ....
....

Personal hygiene: bathe ......   teeth ......
style hair ......   get dressed ......   other ......

Pain Management Strategies:

☐ deep breathing ☐ meditation
☐ visualization ☐ one object focus
☐ calming scents ☐ PMR
☐ rest ☐ music

Something that made me smile:
....
....
Something I am proud of: ....
....
Something I am grateful for: ....
....
Something I am looking forward to: ....
....

Lowest pain level today: 1 2 3 4 5
Highest pain level today: 1 2 3 4 5

Wednesday.........................

Sleep rating: 1 2 3 4 5

Mindset goal: ....
....

Eating goal: ....
....

Personal hygiene: bathe ......   teeth ......
style hair ......   get dressed ......   other ......

Pain Management Strategies:

☐ deep breathing ☐ meditation
☐ visualization ☐ one object focus
☐ calming scents ☐ PMR
☐ rest ☐ music

Something that made me smile:
....
....
Something I am proud of: ....
....
Something I am grateful for: ....
....
Something I am looking forward to: ....
....

Lowest pain level today: 1 2 3 4 5
Highest pain level today: 1 2 3 4 5

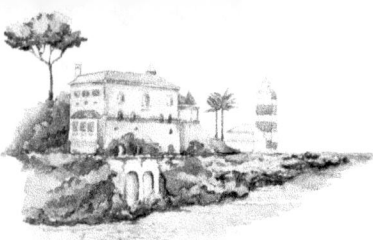

Sleep rating: 1 2 3 4 5

Mindset goal: ....
....

Eating goal: ....
....

Personal hygiene: bathe ......   teeth ......
style hair ......   get dressed ......   other ......

Pain Management Strategies:

- ☐ deep breathing ☐ meditation
- ☐ visualization ☐ one object focus
- ☐ calming scents ☐ PMR
- ☐ rest ☐ music

Something that made me smile:
....
....
Something I am proud of: ....
....
Something I am grateful for: ....
....
Something I am looking forward to: ....
....
....

Lowest pain level today: 1 2 3 4 5
Highest pain level today: 1 2 3 4 5

Friday........................

Sleep rating: 1 2 3 4 5

Mindset goal: ....
....

Eating goal: ....
....

Personal hygiene: bathe ......   teeth ......
style hair ......   get dressed ......   other ......

Pain Management Strategies:

- ☐ deep breathing ☐ meditation
- ☐ visualization ☐ one object focus
- ☐ calming scents ☐ PMR
- ☐ rest ☐ music

Something that made me smile:
....
....
Something I am proud of: ....
....
Something I am grateful for: ....
....
Something I am looking forward to: ....
....
....

Lowest pain level today: 1 2 3 4 5
Highest pain level today: 1 2 3 4 5

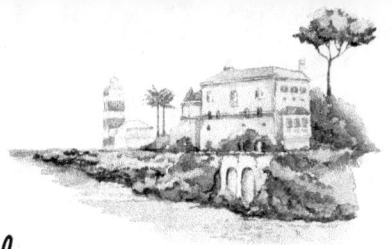

Saturday.......................

Week Thirty-Eight

Sleep rating: 1 2 3 4 5

Mindset goal: ....

....

Eating goal: ....

....

Personal hygiene: bathe ...... teeth ......
style hair ...... get dressed ...... other ......

Pain Management Strategies:

☐ deep breathing ☐ meditation
☐ visualization ☐ one object focus
☐ calming scents ☐ PMR
☐ rest ☐ music

Something that made me smile:

....

....

Something I am proud of: ....

....

Something I am grateful for: ....

....

Something I am looking forward to: ....

....

Lowest pain level today: 1 2 3 4 5
Highest pain level today: 1 2 3 4 5

Sunday.........................

Sleep rating: 1 2 3 4 5

Mindset goal: ....

....

Eating goal: ....

....

Personal hygiene: bathe ...... teeth ......
style hair ...... get dressed ...... other ......

Pain Management Strategies:

☐ deep breathing ☐ meditation
☐ visualization ☐ one object focus
☐ calming scents ☐ PMR
☐ rest ☐ music

Something that made me smile:

....

....

Something I am proud of: ....

....

Something I am grateful for: ....

....

Something I am looking forward to: ....

....

Lowest pain level today: 1 2 3 4 5
Highest pain level today: 1 2 3 4 5

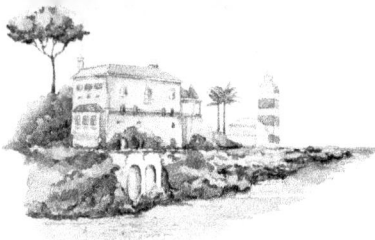

Week Thirty-Nine

Goal for the week: ....
....

Days/Times I will leave the house or change settings: ....
....

When I will interact with friends or family: ....
....

Hobby I will work on: ....

Something new I'll try: ....

Medical tasks to do : ....
....
....

Monday.........................

Sleep rating: 1 2 3 4 5

Mindset goal: ....
....

Eating goal: ....
....

Personal hygiene: bathe ......   teeth ......
style hair ......   get dressed ......   other ......

Pain Management Strategies:

- [ ] deep breathing   [ ] meditation
- [ ] visualization   [ ] one object focus
- [ ] calming scents   [ ] PMR
- [ ] rest   [ ] music

Something that made me smile:
....
....

Something I am proud of: ....
....

Something I am grateful for: ....
....

Something I am looking forward to: ....
....
....

Lowest pain level today: 1 2 3 4 5
Highest pain level today: 1 2 3 4 5

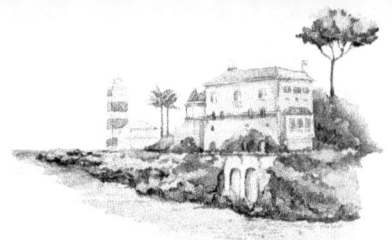

Tuesday............................ *Week Thirty-Nine*

Sleep rating: 1 2 3 4 5

Mindset goal: ....
....

Eating goal: ....
....

Personal hygiene: bathe ......   teeth ......
style hair ......   get dressed ......   other ......

Pain Management Strategies:

☐ deep breathing ☐ meditation
☐ visualization ☐ one object focus
☐ calming scents ☐ PMR
☐ rest ☐ music

Something that made me smile:
....
....
Something I am proud of: ....
....
Something I am grateful for: ....
....
Something I am looking forward to: ....
....
....
Lowest pain level today: 1 2 3 4 5
Highest pain level today: 1 2 3 4 5

Wednesday..........................

Sleep rating: 1 2 3 4 5

Mindset goal: ....
....

Eating goal: ....
....

Personal hygiene: bathe ......   teeth ......
style hair ......   get dressed ......   other ......

Pain Management Strategies:

☐ deep breathing ☐ meditation
☐ visualization ☐ one object focus
☐ calming scents ☐ PMR
☐ rest ☐ music

Something that made me smile:
....
....
Something I am proud of: ....
....
Something I am grateful for: ....
....
Something I am looking forward to: ....
....
....
Lowest pain level today: 1 2 3 4 5
Highest pain level today: 1 2 3 4 5

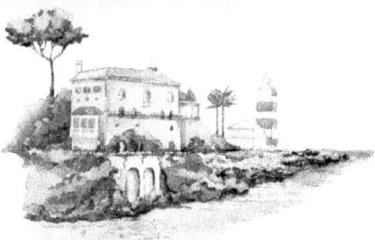

Sleep rating: 1 2 3 4 5

Mindset goal: ....
....

Eating goal: ....
....

Personal hygiene: bathe ...... teeth ......
style hair ...... get dressed ...... other ......

Pain Management Strategies:

☐ deep breathing ☐ meditation
☐ visualization ☐ one object focus
☐ calming scents ☐ PMR
☐ rest ☐ music

Something that made me smile:
....
....

Something I am proud of: ....
....

Something I am grateful for: ....
....

Something I am looking forward to: ....
....
....

Lowest pain level today: 1 2 3 4 5
Highest pain level today: 1 2 3 4 5

Friday........................

Sleep rating: 1 2 3 4 5

Mindset goal: ....
....

Eating goal: ....
....

Personal hygiene: bathe ...... teeth ......
style hair ...... get dressed ...... other ......

Pain Management Strategies:

☐ deep breathing ☐ meditation
☐ visualization ☐ one object focus
☐ calming scents ☐ PMR
☐ rest ☐ music

Something that made me smile:
....
....

Something I am proud of: ....
....

Something I am grateful for: ....
....

Something I am looking forward to: ....
....
....

Lowest pain level today: 1 2 3 4 5
Highest pain level today: 1 2 3 4 5

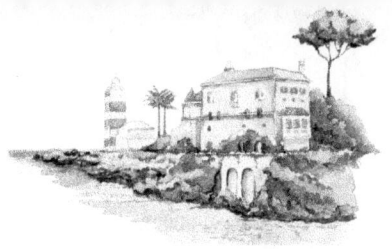

Saturday............................

Week Thirty-Nine

Sleep rating: 1 2 3 4 5

Mindset goal: ....
....

Eating goal: ....
....

Personal hygiene: bathe ...... teeth ......
style hair ...... get dressed ...... other ......

Pain Management Strategies:

☐ deep breathing ☐ meditation
☐ visualization ☐ one object focus
☐ calming scents ☐ PMR
☐ rest ☐ music

Something that made me smile:
....
....

Something I am proud of: ....
....

Something I am grateful for: ....
....

Something I am looking forward to: ....
....

Lowest pain level today: 1 2 3 4 5
Highest pain level today: 1 2 3 4 5

Sunday.........................

Sleep rating: 1 2 3 4 5

Mindset goal: ....
....

Eating goal: ....
....

Personal hygiene: bathe ...... teeth ......
style hair ...... get dressed ...... other ......

Pain Management Strategies:

☐ deep breathing ☐ meditation
☐ visualization ☐ one object focus
☐ calming scents ☐ PMR
☐ rest ☐ music

Something that made me smile:
....
....

Something I am proud of: ....
....

Something I am grateful for: ....
....

Something I am looking forward to: ....
....

Lowest pain level today: 1 2 3 4 5
Highest pain level today: 1 2 3 4 5

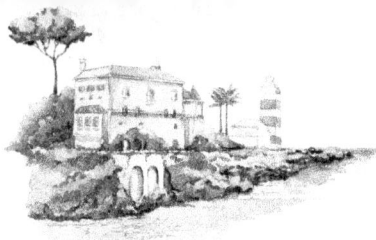

Week Forty

Goal for the week: ....
....

Days/Times I will leave the house or change settings: ....
....

When I will interact with friends or family: ....
....

Hobby I will work on: ....

Something new I'll try: ....

Medical tasks to do : ....
....
....

Monday.........................

Sleep rating: 1 2 3 4 5

Mindset goal: ....
....

Eating goal: ....
....

Personal hygiene: bathe ......   teeth ......
style hair ......   get dressed ......   other ......

Pain Management Strategies:

- [ ] deep breathing
- [ ] visualization
- [ ] calming scents
- [ ] rest
- [ ] meditation
- [ ] one object focus
- [ ] PMR
- [ ] music

Something that made me smile:
....
....

Something I am proud of: ....
....

Something I am grateful for: ....
....

Something I am looking forward to: ....
....
....

Lowest pain level today: 1 2 3 4 5
Highest pain level today: 1 2 3 4 5

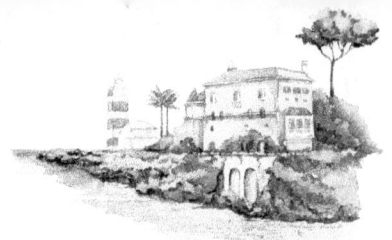

Tuesday.........................

Sleep rating: 1 2 3 4 5

Mindset goal: ....
....

Eating goal: ....
....

Personal hygiene: bathe ...... teeth ......
style hair ...... get dressed ...... other ......

Pain Management Strategies:

☐ deep breathing ☐ meditation
☐ visualization ☐ one object focus
☐ calming scents ☐ PMR
☐ rest ☐ music

Something that made me smile:
....
....

Something I am proud of: ....
....

Something I am grateful for: ....
....

Something I am looking forward to: ....
....

Lowest pain level today: 1 2 3 4 5
Highest pain level today: 1 2 3 4 5

Wednesday.........................

Sleep rating: 1 2 3 4 5

Mindset goal: ....
....

Eating goal: ....
....

Personal hygiene: bathe ...... teeth ......
style hair ...... get dressed ...... other ......

Pain Management Strategies:

☐ deep breathing ☐ meditation
☐ visualization ☐ one object focus
☐ calming scents ☐ PMR
☐ rest ☐ music

Something that made me smile:
....
....

Something I am proud of: ....
....

Something I am grateful for: ....
....

Something I am looking forward to: ....
....

Lowest pain level today: 1 2 3 4 5
Highest pain level today: 1 2 3 4 5

Thursday.....................

Sleep rating: 1 2 3 4 5

Mindset goal: ....
....

Eating goal: ....
....

Personal hygiene: bathe ......   teeth ......
style hair ......   get dressed ......   other ......

Pain Management Strategies:

☐ deep breathing   ☐ meditation
☐ visualization   ☐ one object focus
☐ calming scents   ☐ PMR
☐ rest   ☐ music

Something that made me smile:
....
....

Something I am proud of: ....
....

Something I am grateful for: ....
....

Something I am looking forward to: ....
....
....

Lowest pain level today: 1 2 3 4 5
Highest pain level today: 1 2 3 4 5

Friday..........................

Sleep rating: 1 2 3 4 5

Mindset goal: ....
....

Eating goal: ....
....

Personal hygiene: bathe ......   teeth ......
style hair ......   get dressed ......   other ......

Pain Management Strategies:

☐ deep breathing   ☐ meditation
☐ visualization   ☐ one object focus
☐ calming scents   ☐ PMR
☐ rest   ☐ music

Something that made me smile:
....
....

Something I am proud of: ....
....

Something I am grateful for: ....
....

Something I am looking forward to: ....
....
....

Lowest pain level today: 1 2 3 4 5
Highest pain level today: 1 2 3 4 5

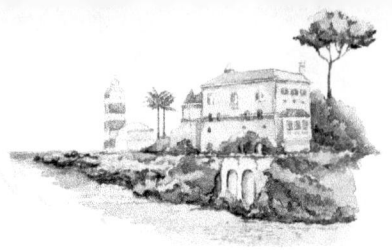

Week Forty

Saturday........................

Sleep rating: 1 2 3 4 5

Mindset goal: ....
....

Eating goal: ....
....

Personal hygiene: bathe ......   teeth ......
style hair ......   get dressed ......   other ......

Pain Management Strategies:

- ☐ deep breathing ☐ meditation
- ☐ visualization ☐ one object focus
- ☐ calming scents ☐ PMR
- ☐ rest ☐ music

Something that made me smile:
....
....

Something I am proud of: ....
....

Something I am grateful for: ....
....

Something I am looking forward to: ....
....
....

Lowest pain level today: 1 2 3 4 5
Highest pain level today: 1 2 3 4 5

Sunday........................

Sleep rating: 1 2 3 4 5

Mindset goal: ....
....

Eating goal: ....
....

Personal hygiene: bathe ......   teeth ......
style hair ......   get dressed ......   other ......

Pain Management Strategies:

- ☐ deep breathing ☐ meditation
- ☐ visualization ☐ one object focus
- ☐ calming scents ☐ PMR
- ☐ rest ☐ music

Something that made me smile:
....
....

Something I am proud of: ....
....

Something I am grateful for: ....
....

Something I am looking forward to: ....
....
....

Lowest pain level today: 1 2 3 4 5
Highest pain level today: 1 2 3 4 5

Monthly Reflection

Think about how your mental health was this month. Did you use the strategies?
When were you your best? Your worst?

....
....
....
....
....
....
....
....
....
....
....
....
....
....
....
....
....
....

Happy Distraction

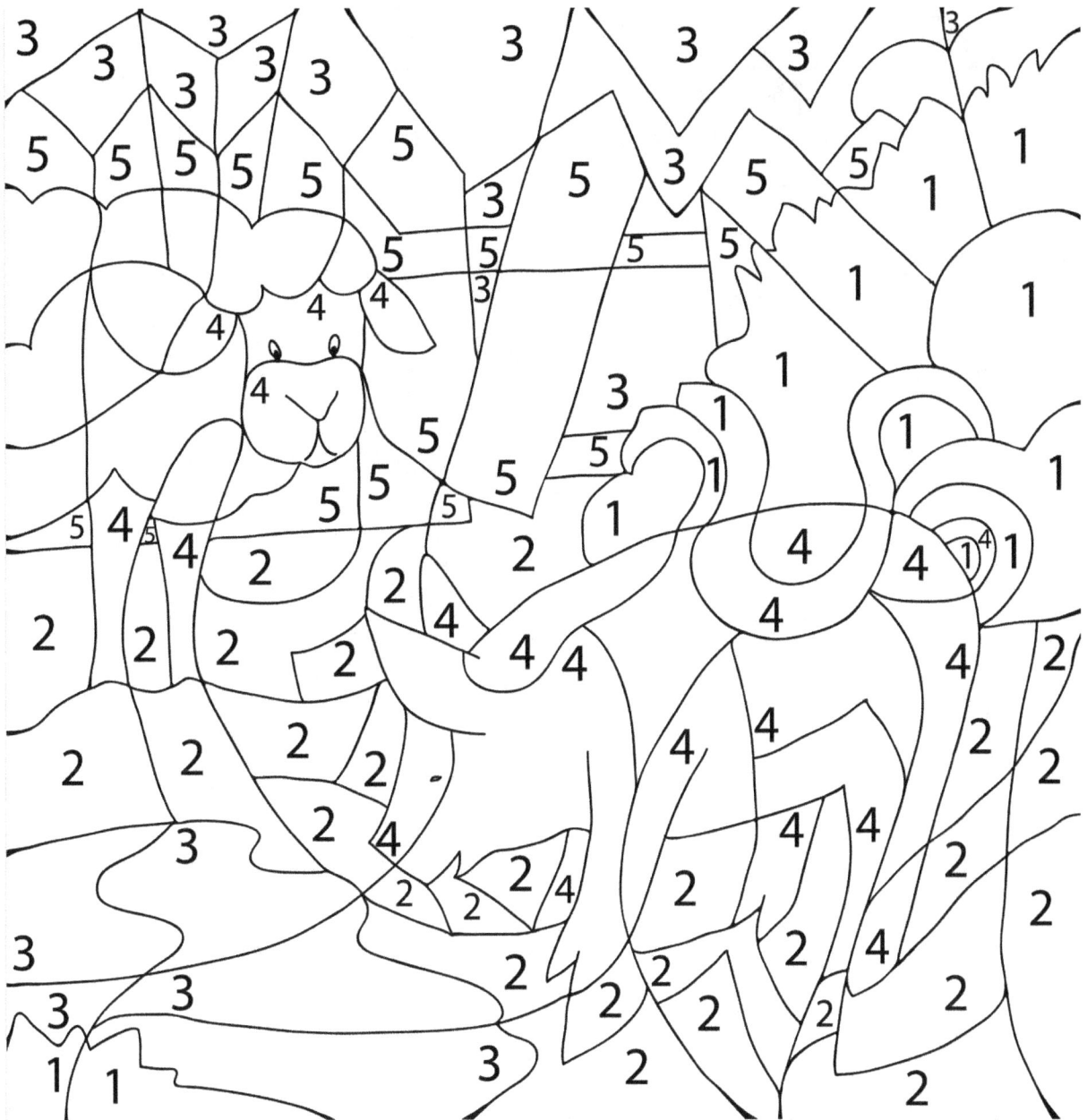

1 = dark green   2 = light green   3 = light blue   4 = pink   5 = brown

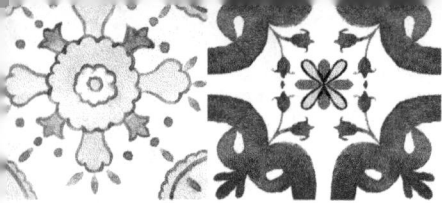

Week Forty-One

Goal for the week: ....
....

Days/Times I will leave the house or change settings: ....
....

When I will interact with friends or family: ....
....

Hobby I will work on: ....

Something new I'll try: ....

Medical tasks to do : ....
....
....

Monday.........................

Sleep rating: 1 2 3 4 5

Mindset goal: ....
....

Eating goal: ....
....

Personal hygiene: bathe ......   teeth ......
style hair ......   get dressed ......   other ......

Pain Management Strategies:

☐ deep breathing ☐ meditation
☐ visualization   ☐ one object focus
☐ calming scents ☐ PMR
☐ rest   ☐ music

Something that made me smile:
....
....

Something I am proud of: ....
....

Something I am grateful for: ....
....

Something I am looking forward to: ....
....
....

Lowest pain level today: 1 2 3 4 5
Highest pain level today: 1 2 3 4 5

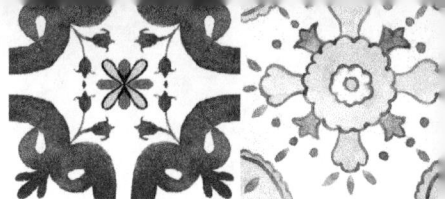

Tuesday...........................

Sleep rating: 1 2 3 4 5

Mindset goal: ....
....

Eating goal: ....
....

Personal hygiene: bathe ...... teeth ......
style hair ...... get dressed ...... other ......

Pain Management Strategies:

☐ deep breathing ☐ meditation
☐ visualization ☐ one object focus
☐ calming scents ☐ PMR
☐ rest ☐ music

Something that made me smile:
....
....

Something I am proud of: ....
....

Something I am grateful for: ....
....

Something I am looking forward to: ....
....

Lowest pain level today: 1 2 3 4 5
Highest pain level today: 1 2 3 4 5

Wednesday...........................

Sleep rating: 1 2 3 4 5

Mindset goal: ....
....

Eating goal: ....
....

Personal hygiene: bathe ...... teeth ......
style hair ...... get dressed ...... other ......

Pain Management Strategies:

☐ deep breathing ☐ meditation
☐ visualization ☐ one object focus
☐ calming scents ☐ PMR
☐ rest ☐ music

Something that made me smile:
....
....

Something I am proud of: ....
....

Something I am grateful for: ....
....

Something I am looking forward to: ....
....

Lowest pain level today: 1 2 3 4 5
Highest pain level today: 1 2 3 4 5

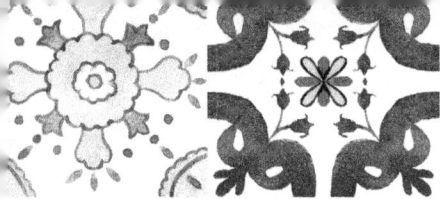

Thursday.....................

Sleep rating: 1 2 3 4 5

Mindset goal: ....

....

Eating goal: ....

....

Personal hygiene: bathe ......   teeth ......
style hair ......   get dressed ......   other ......

Pain Management Strategies:

☐ deep breathing ☐ meditation
☐ visualization ☐ one object focus
☐ calming scents ☐ PMR
☐ rest ☐ music

Something that made me smile:

....

Something I am proud of: ....

....

Something I am grateful for: ....

....

Something I am looking forward to: ....

....

Lowest pain level today: 1 2 3 4 5
Highest pain level today: 1 2 3 4 5

Friday.........................

Sleep rating: 1 2 3 4 5

Mindset goal: ....

....

Eating goal: ....

....

Personal hygiene: bathe ......   teeth ......
style hair ......   get dressed ......   other ......

Pain Management Strategies:

☐ deep breathing ☐ meditation
☐ visualization ☐ one object focus
☐ calming scents ☐ PMR
☐ rest ☐ music

Something that made me smile:

....

Something I am proud of: ....

....

Something I am grateful for: ....

....

Something I am looking forward to: ....

....

Lowest pain level today: 1 2 3 4 5
Highest pain level today: 1 2 3 4 5

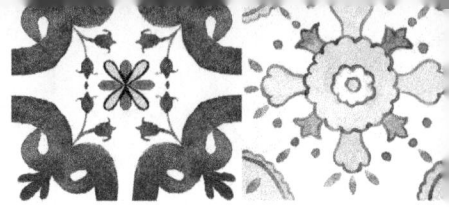

Saturday........................

Sleep rating: 1 2 3 4 5

Mindset goal: ....
....

Eating goal: ....
....

Personal hygiene: bathe ...... teeth ......
style hair ...... get dressed ...... other ......

Pain Management Strategies:

☐ deep breathing ☐ meditation
☐ visualization ☐ one object focus
☐ calming scents ☐ PMR
☐ rest ☐ music

Something that made me smile:
....
....
Something I am proud of: ....
....
Something I am grateful for: ....
....
....
Something I am looking forward to: ....
....
....
Lowest pain level today: 1 2 3 4 5
Highest pain level today: 1 2 3 4 5

Sunday.........................

Sleep rating: 1 2 3 4 5

Mindset goal: ....
....

Eating goal: ....
....

Personal hygiene: bathe ...... teeth ......
style hair ...... get dressed ...... other ......

Pain Management Strategies:

☐ deep breathing ☐ meditation
☐ visualization ☐ one object focus
☐ calming scents ☐ PMR
☐ rest ☐ music

Something that made me smile:
....
....
Something I am proud of: ....
....
Something I am grateful for: ....
....
....
Something I am looking forward to: ....
....
....
Lowest pain level today: 1 2 3 4 5
Highest pain level today: 1 2 3 4 5

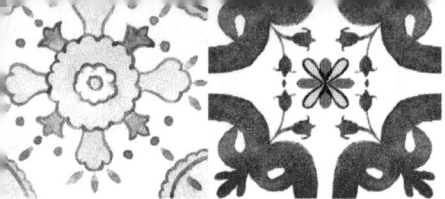

Week Forty-Two

Goal for the week: ....
....

Days/Times I will leave the house or change settings: ....
....

When I will interact with friends or family: ....
....

Hobby I will work on: ....

Something new I'll try: ....

Medical tasks to do : ....
....
....

Monday...........................

Sleep rating: 1 2 3 4 5

Mindset goal: ....
....

Eating goal: ....
....

Personal hygiene: bathe ......   teeth ......
style hair ......   get dressed ......   other ......

Pain Management Strategies:

- [ ] deep breathing [ ] meditation
- [ ] visualization [ ] one object focus
- [ ] calming scents [ ] PMR
- [ ] rest [ ] music

Something that made me smile:
....
....

Something I am proud of: ....
....

Something I am grateful for: ....
....

Something I am looking forward to: ....
....
....

Lowest pain level today: 1 2 3 4 5
Highest pain level today: 1 2 3 4 5

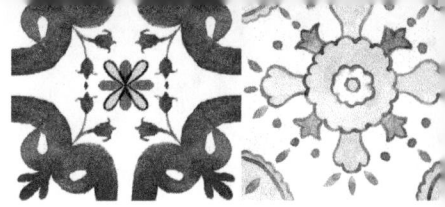

Sleep rating: 1 2 3 4 5

Mindset goal: ....
....

Eating goal: ....
....

Personal hygiene: bathe ...... teeth ......
style hair ...... get dressed ...... other ......

Pain Management Strategies:

☐ deep breathing ☐ meditation
☐ visualization ☐ one object focus
☐ calming scents ☐ PMR
☐ rest ☐ music

Something that made me smile:
....
....
Something I am proud of: ....
....
Something I am grateful for: ....
....
Something I am looking forward to: ....
....

Lowest pain level today: 1 2 3 4 5
Highest pain level today: 1 2 3 4 5

Wednesday..........................

Sleep rating: 1 2 3 4 5

Mindset goal: ....
....

Eating goal: ....
....

Personal hygiene: bathe ...... teeth ......
style hair ...... get dressed ...... other ......

Pain Management Strategies:

☐ deep breathing ☐ meditation
☐ visualization ☐ one object focus
☐ calming scents ☐ PMR
☐ rest ☐ music

Something that made me smile:
....
....
Something I am proud of: ....
....
Something I am grateful for: ....
....
Something I am looking forward to: ....
....

Lowest pain level today: 1 2 3 4 5
Highest pain level today: 1 2 3 4 5

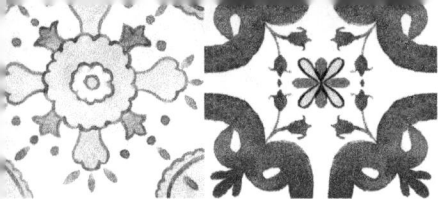

Sleep rating: 1 2 3 4 5

Mindset goal: ....
....

Eating goal: ....
....

Personal hygiene: bathe ...... teeth ......
style hair ...... get dressed ...... other ......

Pain Management Strategies:

☐ deep breathing ☐ meditation
☐ visualization ☐ one object focus
☐ calming scents ☐ PMR
☐ rest ☐ music

Something that made me smile:
....
....

Something I am proud of: ....

Something I am grateful for: ....

Something I am looking forward to: ....

Lowest pain level today: 1 2 3 4 5
Highest pain level today: 1 2 3 4 5

Friday........................

Sleep rating: 1 2 3 4 5

Mindset goal: ....
....

Eating goal: ....
....

Personal hygiene: bathe ...... teeth ......
style hair ...... get dressed ...... other ......

Pain Management Strategies:

☐ deep breathing ☐ meditation
☐ visualization ☐ one object focus
☐ calming scents ☐ PMR
☐ rest ☐ music

Something that made me smile:
....
....

Something I am proud of: ....

Something I am grateful for: ....

Something I am looking forward to: ....

Lowest pain level today: 1 2 3 4 5
Highest pain level today: 1 2 3 4 5

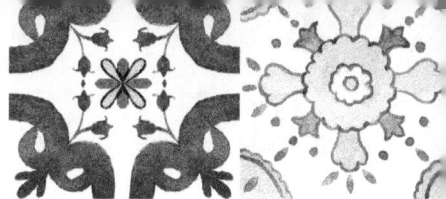

Week Forty-Two

Saturday......................

Sleep rating: 1 2 3 4 5

Mindset goal: ....
....

Eating goal: ....
....

Personal hygiene: bathe ...... teeth ......
style hair ...... get dressed ...... other ......

Pain Management Strategies:

- [ ] deep breathing   [ ] meditation
- [ ] visualization   [ ] one object focus
- [ ] calming scents   [ ] PMR
- [ ] rest   [ ] music

Something that made me smile:
....
....

Something I am proud of: ....
....

Something I am grateful for: ....
....

Something I am looking forward to: ....
....

Lowest pain level today: 1 2 3 4 5
Highest pain level today: 1 2 3 4 5

Sunday........................

Sleep rating: 1 2 3 4 5

Mindset goal: ....
....

Eating goal: ....
....

Personal hygiene: bathe ...... teeth ......
style hair ...... get dressed ...... other ......

Pain Management Strategies:

- [ ] deep breathing   [ ] meditation
- [ ] visualization   [ ] one object focus
- [ ] calming scents   [ ] PMR
- [ ] rest   [ ] music

Something that made me smile:
....
....

Something I am proud of: ....
....

Something I am grateful for: ....
....

Something I am looking forward to: ....
....

Lowest pain level today: 1 2 3 4 5
Highest pain level today: 1 2 3 4 5

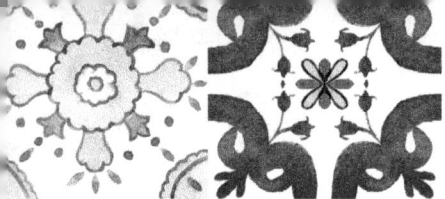

Week Forty-Three

Goal for the week: ....
....

Days/Times I will leave the house or change settings: ....
....

When I will interact with friends or family: ....
....

Hobby I will work on: ....

Something new I'll try: ....

Medical tasks to do : ....
....
....

Monday.........................

Sleep rating: 1 2 3 4 5

Mindset goal: ....
....

Eating goal: ....
....

Personal hygiene: bathe ...... teeth ......
style hair ...... get dressed ...... other ......

Pain Management Strategies:

☐ deep breathing ☐ meditation
☐ visualization ☐ one object focus
☐ calming scents ☐ PMR
☐ rest ☐ music

Something that made me smile: ....
....
....

Something I am proud of: ....
....

Something I am grateful for: ....
....

Something I am looking forward to: ....
....
....

Lowest pain level today: 1 2 3 4 5
Highest pain level today: 1 2 3 4 5

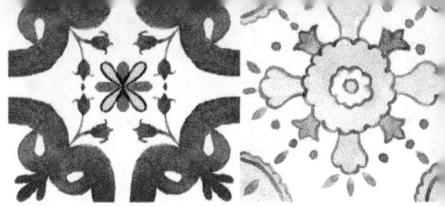

Tuesday...................

Sleep rating: 1 2 3 4 5

Mindset goal: ....
....

Eating goal: ....
....

Personal hygiene: bathe ...... teeth ......
style hair ...... get dressed ...... other ......

Pain Management Strategies:

☐ deep breathing ☐ meditation
☐ visualization ☐ one object focus
☐ calming scents ☐ PMR
☐ rest ☐ music

Something that made me smile:
....
....
Something I am proud of: ....
....
Something I am grateful for: ....
....
Something I am looking forward to: ....
....
Lowest pain level today: 1 2 3 4 5
Highest pain level today: 1 2 3 4 5

Wednesday.........................

Sleep rating: 1 2 3 4 5

Mindset goal: ....
....

Eating goal: ....
....

Personal hygiene: bathe ...... teeth ......
style hair ...... get dressed ...... other ......

Pain Management Strategies:

☐ deep breathing ☐ meditation
☐ visualization ☐ one object focus
☐ calming scents ☐ PMR
☐ rest ☐ music

Something that made me smile:
....
....
Something I am proud of: ....
....
Something I am grateful for: ....
....
....
Something I am looking forward to: ....
....
....
Lowest pain level today: 1 2 3 4 5
Highest pain level today: 1 2 3 4 5

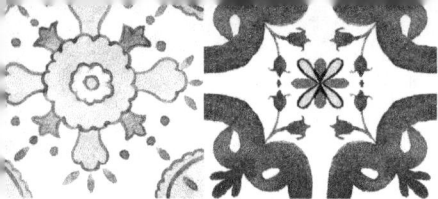

Thursday........................

Sleep rating: 1 2 3 4 5

Mindset goal: ....
....

Eating goal: ....
....

Personal hygiene: bathe ...... teeth ......
style hair ...... get dressed ...... other ......

Pain Management Strategies:

- [ ] deep breathing [ ] meditation
- [ ] visualization [ ] one object focus
- [ ] calming scents [ ] PMR
- [ ] rest [ ] music

Something that made me smile:
....
....

Something I am proud of: ....
....

Something I am grateful for: ....
....

Something I am looking forward to: ....
....
....

Lowest pain level today: 1 2 3 4 5
Highest pain level today: 1 2 3 4 5

Friday.........................

Sleep rating: 1 2 3 4 5

Mindset goal: ....
....

Eating goal: ....
....

Personal hygiene: bathe ...... teeth ......
style hair ...... get dressed ...... other ......

Pain Management Strategies:

- [ ] deep breathing [ ] meditation
- [ ] visualization [ ] one object focus
- [ ] calming scents [ ] PMR
- [ ] rest [ ] music

Something that made me smile:
....
....

Something I am proud of: ....
....

Something I am grateful for: ....
....

Something I am looking forward to: ....
....
....

Lowest pain level today: 1 2 3 4 5
Highest pain level today: 1 2 3 4 5

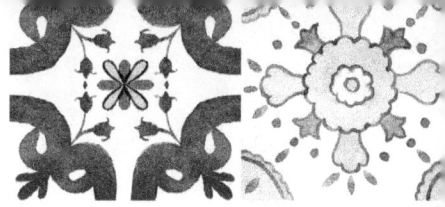

Sleep rating: 1 2 3 4 5

Mindset goal: ....
....

Eating goal: ....
....

Personal hygiene: bathe ...... teeth ......
style hair ...... get dressed ...... other ......

Pain Management Strategies:

☐ deep breathing ☐ meditation
☐ visualization ☐ one object focus
☐ calming scents ☐ PMR
☐ rest ☐ music

Something that made me smile:
....
....
Something I am proud of: ....
....
Something I am grateful for: ....
....
Something I am looking forward to: ....
....

Lowest pain level today: 1 2 3 4 5
Highest pain level today: 1 2 3 4 5

Sunday........................

Sleep rating: 1 2 3 4 5

Mindset goal: ....
....

Eating goal: ....
....

Personal hygiene: bathe ...... teeth ......
style hair ...... get dressed ...... other ......

Pain Management Strategies:

☐ deep breathing ☐ meditation
☐ visualization ☐ one object focus
☐ calming scents ☐ PMR
☐ rest ☐ music

Something that made me smile:
....
....
Something I am proud of: ....
....
Something I am grateful for: ....
....
Something I am looking forward to: ....
....

Lowest pain level today: 1 2 3 4 5
Highest pain level today: 1 2 3 4 5

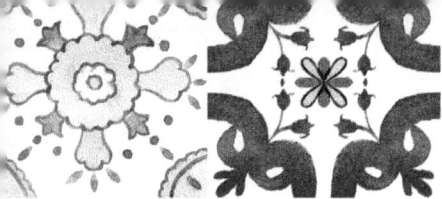

Week Forty-Four

Goal for the week: ....
....

Days/Times I will leave the house or change settings: ....
....

When I will interact with friends or family: ....
....

Hobby I will work on: ....

Something new I'll try: ....

Medical tasks to do : ....
....
....

Monday........................

Sleep rating: 1 2 3 4 5

Mindset goal: ....
....

Eating goal: ....
....

Personal hygiene: bathe ......   teeth ......
style hair ......   get dressed ......   other ......

Pain Management Strategies:

- [ ] deep breathing [ ] meditation
- [ ] visualization   [ ] one object focus
- [ ] calming scents [ ] PMR
- [ ] rest   [ ] music

Something that made me smile:
....
....

Something I am proud of: ....
....

Something I am grateful for: ....
....

Something I am looking forward to: ....
....
....

Lowest pain level today: 1 2 3 4 5
Highest pain level today: 1 2 3 4 5

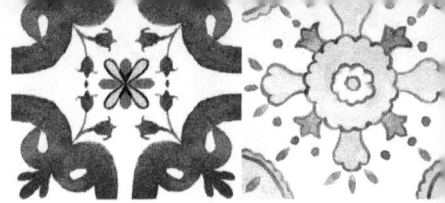

Week Forty-Four

Tuesday...................

Sleep rating: 1 2 3 4 5

Mindset goal: ....
....

Eating goal: ....
....

Personal hygiene: bathe ......   teeth ......
style hair ......   get dressed ......   other ......

Pain Management Strategies:

☐ deep breathing ☐ meditation
☐ visualization ☐ one object focus
☐ calming scents ☐ PMR
☐ rest ☐ music

Something that made me smile:
....
....

Something I am proud of: ....
....

Something I am grateful for: ....
....

Something I am looking forward to: ....
....

Lowest pain level today: 1 2 3 4 5
Highest pain level today: 1 2 3 4 5

Wednesday.........................

Sleep rating: 1 2 3 4 5

Mindset goal: ....
....

Eating goal: ....
....

Personal hygiene: bathe ......   teeth ......
style hair ......   get dressed ......   other ......

Pain Management Strategies:

☐ deep breathing ☐ meditation
☐ visualization ☐ one object focus
☐ calming scents ☐ PMR
☐ rest ☐ music

Something that made me smile:
....
....

Something I am proud of: ....
....

Something I am grateful for: ....
....

Something I am looking forward to: ....
....

Lowest pain level today: 1 2 3 4 5
Highest pain level today: 1 2 3 4 5

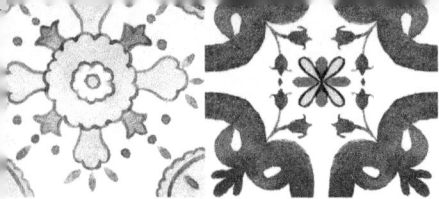

Thursday.....................

Sleep rating: 1 2 3 4 5

Mindset goal: ....

....

Eating goal: ....

....

Personal hygiene: bathe ......   teeth ......
style hair ......   get dressed ......   other ......

Pain Management Strategies:

☐ deep breathing   ☐ meditation
☐ visualization   ☐ one object focus
☐ calming scents   ☐ PMR
☐ rest   ☐ music

Something that made me smile:
....
....
Something I am proud of: ....
....
Something I am grateful for: ....
....
Something I am looking forward to: ....
....
....
Lowest pain level today: 1 2 3 4 5
Highest pain level today: 1 2 3 4 5

Friday.........................

Sleep rating: 1 2 3 4 5

Mindset goal: ....

....

Eating goal: ....

....

Personal hygiene: bathe ......   teeth ......
style hair ......   get dressed ......   other ......

Pain Management Strategies:

☐ deep breathing   ☐ meditation
☐ visualization   ☐ one object focus
☐ calming scents   ☐ PMR
☐ rest   ☐ music

Something that made me smile:
....
....
Something I am proud of: ....
....
Something I am grateful for: ....
....
Something I am looking forward to: ....
....
....
Lowest pain level today: 1 2 3 4 5
Highest pain level today: 1 2 3 4 5

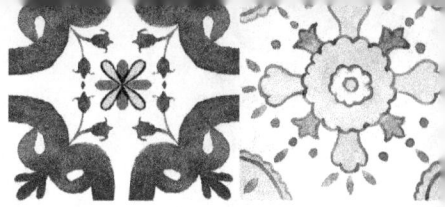

Saturday........................

Sleep rating: 1 2 3 4 5

Mindset goal: ....
....

Eating goal: ....
....

Personal hygiene: bathe ......   teeth ......
style hair ......   get dressed ......   other ......

Pain Management Strategies:

- [ ] deep breathing
- [ ] visualization
- [ ] calming scents
- [ ] rest
- [ ] meditation
- [ ] one object focus
- [ ] PMR
- [ ] music

Something that made me smile:
....
....

Something I am proud of: ....
....

Something I am grateful for: ....
....

Something I am looking forward to: ....
....
....

Lowest pain level today: 1 2 3 4 5
Highest pain level today: 1 2 3 4 5

Sunday........................

Sleep rating: 1 2 3 4 5

Mindset goal: ....
....

Eating goal: ....
....

Personal hygiene: bathe ......   teeth ......
style hair ......   get dressed ......   other ......

Pain Management Strategies:

- [ ] deep breathing
- [ ] visualization
- [ ] calming scents
- [ ] rest
- [ ] meditation
- [ ] one object focus
- [ ] PMR
- [ ] music

Something that made me smile:
....
....

Something I am proud of: ....
....

Something I am grateful for: ....
....

Something I am looking forward to: ....
....
....

Lowest pain level today: 1 2 3 4 5
Highest pain level today: 1 2 3 4 5

Monthly Reflection

Think about how your mental health was this month. Did you use the strategies?
When were you your best? Your worst?

....

....

....

....

....

....

....

....

....

....

....

....

....

....

....

....

....

....

Happy Distraction

Word Jumble: Unscramble the letters to create a cleaning-related word or phrase.

TRENDTEEG ....

UCUMAV ....

LOTTIE HURBS ....

WELMID ....

BRICSNUBG ....

ESTRUD ....

SLIPOH ....

GIMAC ASERRE ....

CRETLUT ....

DINTYGI ....

HARDSEHSWI ....

WOLELY EGOSLV ....

XIWDEN ....

OGNEPS ....

GOZIRENA ....

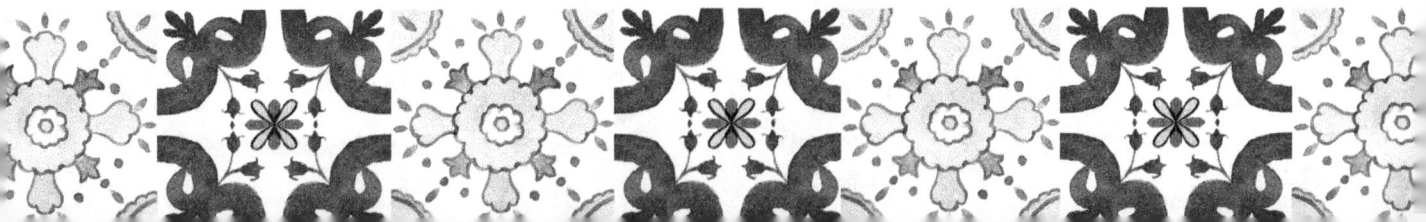

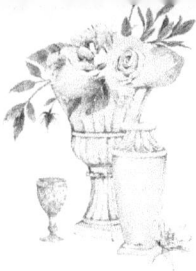

Week Forty-Five

Goal for the week: ....
....

Days/Times I will leave the house or change settings: ....
....

When I will interact with friends or family: ....
....

Hobby I will work on: ....

Something new I'll try: ....

Medical tasks to do : ....
....
....

Monday........................

Sleep rating: 1 2 3 4 5

Mindset goal: ....
....

Eating goal: ....
....

Personal hygiene: bathe ......   teeth ......
style hair ......   get dressed ......   other ......

Pain Management Strategies:

- [ ] deep breathing
- [ ] visualization
- [ ] calming scents
- [ ] rest
- [ ] meditation
- [ ] one object focus
- [ ] PMR
- [ ] music

Something that made me smile:
....
....

Something I am proud of: ....
....

Something I am grateful for: ....
....

Something I am looking forward to: ....
....
....

Lowest pain level today: 1 2 3 4 5
Highest pain level today: 1 2 3 4 5

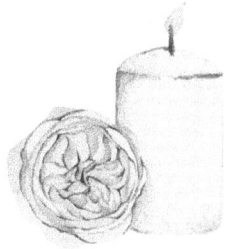

Week Forty-Five

Tuesday....................

Sleep rating: 1 2 3 4 5

Mindset goal: ....
....

Eating goal: ....
....

Personal hygiene: bathe ......   teeth ......
style hair ......   get dressed ......   other ......

Pain Management Strategies:

☐ deep breathing   ☐ meditation
☐ visualization   ☐ one object focus
☐ calming scents   ☐ PMR
☐ rest   ☐ music

Something that made me smile:
....

Something I am proud of: ....
....

Something I am grateful for: ....
....

Something I am looking forward to: ....
....

Lowest pain level today: 1 2 3 4 5
Highest pain level today: 1 2 3 4 5

Wednesday........................

Sleep rating: 1 2 3 4 5

Mindset goal: ....
....

Eating goal: ....
....

Personal hygiene: bathe ......   teeth ......
style hair ......   get dressed ......   other ......

Pain Management Strategies:

☐ deep breathing   ☐ meditation
☐ visualization   ☐ one object focus
☐ calming scents   ☐ PMR
☐ rest   ☐ music

Something that made me smile:
....
....

Something I am proud of: ....
....

Something I am grateful for: ....
....

Something I am looking forward to: ....
....

Lowest pain level today: 1 2 3 4 5
Highest pain level today: 1 2 3 4 5

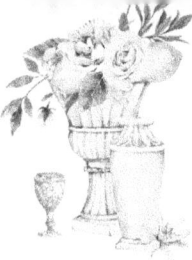

Sleep rating: 1 2 3 4 5

Mindset goal: ....
....

Eating goal: ....
....

Personal hygiene: bathe ...... teeth ......
style hair ...... get dressed ...... other ......

Pain Management Strategies:

☐ deep breathing ☐ meditation
☐ visualization ☐ one object focus
☐ calming scents ☐ PMR
☐ rest ☐ music

Something that made me smile:
....
....

Something I am proud of: ....
....

Something I am grateful for: ....
....

Something I am looking forward to: ....
....
....

Lowest pain level today: 1 2 3 4 5
Highest pain level today: 1 2 3 4 5

Friday..........................

Sleep rating: 1 2 3 4 5

Mindset goal: ....
....

Eating goal: ....
....

Personal hygiene: bathe ...... teeth ......
style hair ...... get dressed ...... other ......

Pain Management Strategies:

☐ deep breathing ☐ meditation
☐ visualization ☐ one object focus
☐ calming scents ☐ PMR
☐ rest ☐ music

Something that made me smile:
....
....

Something I am proud of: ....
....

Something I am grateful for: ....
....

Something I am looking forward to: ....
....
....

Lowest pain level today: 1 2 3 4 5
Highest pain level today: 1 2 3 4 5

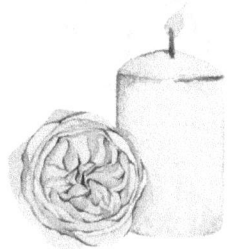

Saturday...................... *Week Forty-Five*

Sleep rating: 1 2 3 4 5

Mindset goal: ....
....

Eating goal: ....
....

Personal hygiene: bathe ......   teeth ......
style hair ......   get dressed ......   other ......

Pain Management Strategies:

☐ deep breathing ☐ meditation
☐ visualization   ☐ one object focus
☐ calming scents ☐ PMR
☐ rest   ☐ music

Something that made me smile:
....
....
Something I am proud of: ....
....
Something I am grateful for: ....
....
Something I am looking forward to: ....
....

Lowest pain level today: 1 2 3 4 5
Highest pain level today: 1 2 3 4 5

Sunday........................

Sleep rating: 1 2 3 4 5

Mindset goal: ....
....

Eating goal: ....
....

Personal hygiene: bathe ......   teeth ......
style hair ......   get dressed ......   other ......

Pain Management Strategies:

☐ deep breathing ☐ meditation
☐ visualization   ☐ one object focus
☐ calming scents ☐ PMR
☐ rest   ☐ music

Something that made me smile:
....
....
Something I am proud of: ....
....
Something I am grateful for: ....
....
Something I am looking forward to: ....
....

Lowest pain level today: 1 2 3 4 5
Highest pain level today: 1 2 3 4 5

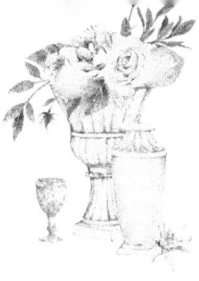

Week Forty-Six

Goal for the week: ....
....

Days/Times I will leave the house or change settings: ....
....

When I will interact with friends or family: ....
....

Hobby I will work on: ....

Something new I'll try: ....

Medical tasks to do : ....
....
....

Monday........................

Sleep rating: 1 2 3 4 5

Mindset goal: ....
....

Eating goal: ....
....

Personal hygiene: bathe ......   teeth ......
style hair ......   get dressed ......   other ......

Pain Management Strategies:

☐ deep breathing ☐ meditation
☐ visualization ☐ one object focus
☐ calming scents ☐ PMR
☐ rest ☐ music

Something that made me smile:
....
....
Something I am proud of: ....
....
Something I am grateful for: ....
....
Something I am looking forward to: ....
....
....
Lowest pain level today: 1 2 3 4 5
Highest pain level today: 1 2 3 4 5

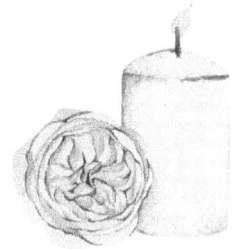

Week Forty-Six

Tuesday.....................

Sleep rating: 1 2 3 4 5

Mindset goal: ....
....

Eating goal: ....
....

Personal hygiene: bathe ...... teeth ......
style hair ...... get dressed ...... other ......

Pain Management Strategies:

☐ deep breathing ☐ meditation
☐ visualization ☐ one object focus
☐ calming scents ☐ PMR
☐ rest ☐ music

Something that made me smile:
....
....

Something I am proud of: ....
....
....

Something I am grateful for: ....
....
....

Something I am looking forward to: ....
....
....

Lowest pain level today: 1 2 3 4 5
Highest pain level today: 1 2 3 4 5

Wednesday........................

Sleep rating: 1 2 3 4 5

Mindset goal: ....
....

Eating goal: ....
....

Personal hygiene: bathe ...... teeth ......
style hair ...... get dressed ...... other ......

Pain Management Strategies:

☐ deep breathing ☐ meditation
☐ visualization ☐ one object focus
☐ calming scents ☐ PMR
☐ rest ☐ music

Something that made me smile:
....
....

Something I am proud of: ....
....
....

Something I am grateful for: ....
....
....

Something I am looking forward to: ....
....
....

Lowest pain level today: 1 2 3 4 5
Highest pain level today: 1 2 3 4 5

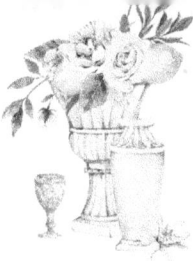

Thursday.....................

Sleep rating: 1 2 3 4 5

Mindset goal: ....
....

Eating goal: ....
....

Personal hygiene: bathe ......   teeth ......
style hair ......   get dressed ......   other ......

Pain Management Strategies:

- ☐ deep breathing   ☐ meditation
- ☐ visualization   ☐ one object focus
- ☐ calming scents   ☐ PMR
- ☐ rest   ☐ music

Something that made me smile:
....
....

Something I am proud of: ....
....

Something I am grateful for: ....
....

Something I am looking forward to: ....
....
....

Lowest pain level today: 1 2 3 4 5
Highest pain level today: 1 2 3 4 5

Friday........................

Sleep rating: 1 2 3 4 5

Mindset goal: ....
....

Eating goal: ....
....

Personal hygiene: bathe ......   teeth ......
style hair ......   get dressed ......   other ......

Pain Management Strategies:

- ☐ deep breathing   ☐ meditation
- ☐ visualization   ☐ one object focus
- ☐ calming scents   ☐ PMR
- ☐ rest   ☐ music

Something that made me smile:
....
....

Something I am proud of: ....
....

Something I am grateful for: ....
....

Something I am looking forward to: ....
....
....

Lowest pain level today: 1 2 3 4 5
Highest pain level today: 1 2 3 4 5

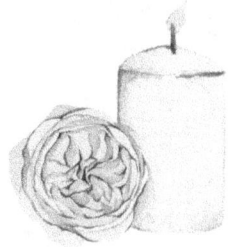

Week Forty-Six

Saturday.....................

Sleep rating: 1 2 3 4 5

Mindset goal: ....
....

Eating goal: ....
....

Personal hygiene: bathe ......   teeth ......
style hair ......   get dressed ......   other ......

Pain Management Strategies:

☐ deep breathing   ☐ meditation
☐ visualization   ☐ one object focus
☐ calming scents   ☐ PMR
☐ rest   ☐ music

Something that made me smile:
....
....
Something I am proud of: ....
....
....
Something I am grateful for: ....
....
....
Something I am looking forward to: ....
....
....
Lowest pain level today: 1 2 3 4 5
Highest pain level today: 1 2 3 4 5

Sunday........................

Sleep rating: 1 2 3 4 5

Mindset goal: ....
....

Eating goal: ....
....

Personal hygiene: bathe ......   teeth ......
style hair ......   get dressed ......   other ......

Pain Management Strategies:

☐ deep breathing   ☐ meditation
☐ visualization   ☐ one object focus
☐ calming scents   ☐ PMR
☐ rest   ☐ music

Something that made me smile:
....
....
Something I am proud of: ....
....
....
Something I am grateful for: ....
....
....
Something I am looking forward to: ....
....
....
Lowest pain level today: 1 2 3 4 5
Highest pain level today: 1 2 3 4 5

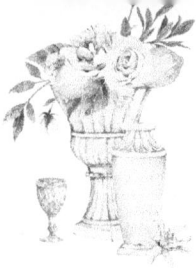

Week Forty-Seven

Goal for the week: ....
....

Days/Times I will leave the house or change settings: ....
....

When I will interact with friends or family: ....
....

Hobby I will work on: ....

Something new I'll try: ....

Medical tasks to do : ....
....
....

Monday.......................

Sleep rating: 1 2 3 4 5

Mindset goal: ....
....

Eating goal: ....
....

Personal hygiene: bathe ......   teeth ......
style hair ......   get dressed ......   other ......

Pain Management Strategies:

☐ deep breathing ☐ meditation
☐ visualization   ☐ one object focus
☐ calming scents ☐ PMR
☐ rest   ☐ music

Something that made me smile:
....
....

Something I am proud of: ....
....

Something I am grateful for: ....
....

Something I am looking forward to: ....
....
....

Lowest pain level today: 1 2 3 4 5
Highest pain level today: 1 2 3 4 5

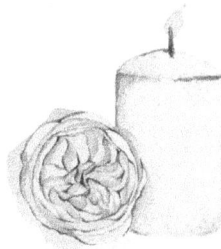

Week Forty-Seven

Tuesday ....

Sleep rating: 1 2 3 4 5

Mindset goal: ....
....

Eating goal: ....
....

Personal hygiene: bathe ...... teeth ......
style hair ...... get dressed ...... other ......

Pain Management Strategies:

- ☐ deep breathing ☐ meditation
- ☐ visualization ☐ one object focus
- ☐ calming scents ☐ PMR
- ☐ rest ☐ music

Something that made me smile:
....
....
Something I am proud of: ....
....
Something I am grateful for: ....
....
Something I am looking forward to: ....
....
....

Lowest pain level today: 1 2 3 4 5
Highest pain level today: 1 2 3 4 5

Wednesday ....

Sleep rating: 1 2 3 4 5

Mindset goal: ....
....

Eating goal: ....
....

Personal hygiene: bathe ...... teeth ......
style hair ...... get dressed ...... other ......

Pain Management Strategies:

- ☐ deep breathing ☐ meditation
- ☐ visualization ☐ one object focus
- ☐ calming scents ☐ PMR
- ☐ rest ☐ music

Something that made me smile:
....
....
Something I am proud of: ....
....
Something I am grateful for: ....
....
Something I am looking forward to: ....
....
....

Lowest pain level today: 1 2 3 4 5
Highest pain level today: 1 2 3 4 5

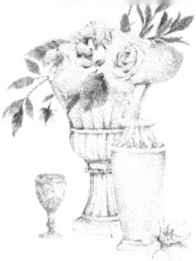

Sleep rating: 1 2 3 4 5

Mindset goal: ....
....

Eating goal: ....
....

Personal hygiene: bathe ...... teeth ......
style hair ...... get dressed ...... other ......

Pain Management Strategies:

☐ deep breathing ☐ meditation
☐ visualization ☐ one object focus
☐ calming scents ☐ PMR
☐ rest ☐ music

Something that made me smile:
....
....
Something I am proud of: ....
....
Something I am grateful for: ....
....
Something I am looking forward to: ....
....
....

Lowest pain level today: 1 2 3 4 5
Highest pain level today: 1 2 3 4 5

Friday........................

Sleep rating: 1 2 3 4 5

Mindset goal: ....
....

Eating goal: ....
....

Personal hygiene: bathe ...... teeth ......
style hair ...... get dressed ...... other ......

Pain Management Strategies:

☐ deep breathing ☐ meditation
☐ visualization ☐ one object focus
☐ calming scents ☐ PMR
☐ rest ☐ music

Something that made me smile:
....
....
Something I am proud of: ....
....
Something I am grateful for: ....
....
Something I am looking forward to: ....
....
....

Lowest pain level today: 1 2 3 4 5
Highest pain level today: 1 2 3 4 5

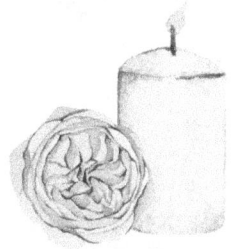

Saturday ....

Week Forty-Seven

Sleep rating: 1 2 3 4 5

Mindset goal: ....

....

Eating goal: ....

....

Personal hygiene: bathe ...... teeth ......
style hair ...... get dressed ...... other ......

Pain Management Strategies:

- [ ] deep breathing
- [ ] visualization
- [ ] calming scents
- [ ] rest
- [ ] meditation
- [ ] one object focus
- [ ] PMR
- [ ] music

Something that made me smile:

....

....

Something I am proud of: ....

....

Something I am grateful for: ....

....

Something I am looking forward to: ....

....

Lowest pain level today: 1 2 3 4 5
Highest pain level today: 1 2 3 4 5

Sunday ....

Sleep rating: 1 2 3 4 5

Mindset goal: ....

....

Eating goal: ....

....

Personal hygiene: bathe ...... teeth ......
style hair ...... get dressed ...... other ......

Pain Management Strategies:

- [ ] deep breathing
- [ ] visualization
- [ ] calming scents
- [ ] rest
- [ ] meditation
- [ ] one object focus
- [ ] PMR
- [ ] music

Something that made me smile:

....

....

Something I am proud of: ....

....

Something I am grateful for: ....

....

Something I am looking forward to: ....

....

Lowest pain level today: 1 2 3 4 5
Highest pain level today: 1 2 3 4 5

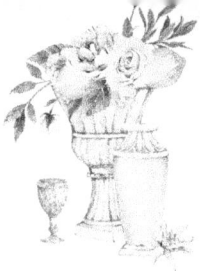

Week Forty-Eight

Goal for the week: ....
....

Days/Times I will leave the house or change settings: ....
....

When I will interact with friends or family: ....
....

Hobby I will work on: ....

Something new I'll try: ....

Medical tasks to do : ....
....
....

Monday.......................

Sleep rating: 1 2 3 4 5

Mindset goal: ....
....

Eating goal: ....
....

Personal hygiene: bathe ......   teeth ......
style hair ......   get dressed ......   other ......

Pain Management Strategies:

- [ ] deep breathing [ ] meditation
- [ ] visualization [ ] one object focus
- [ ] calming scents [ ] PMR
- [ ] rest [ ] music

Something that made me smile:
....
....
Something I am proud of: ....
....
Something I am grateful for: ....
....
Something I am looking forward to: ....
....
....
Lowest pain level today: 1 2 3 4 5
Highest pain level today: 1 2 3 4 5

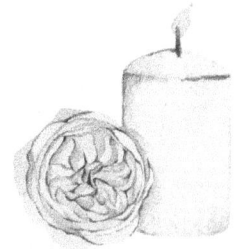

Sleep rating: 1 2 3 4 5

Mindset goal: ....
....

Eating goal: ....
....

Personal hygiene: bathe ...... teeth ......
style hair ...... get dressed ...... other ......

Pain Management Strategies:

- [ ] deep breathing [ ] meditation
- [ ] visualization [ ] one object focus
- [ ] calming scents [ ] PMR
- [ ] rest [ ] music

Something that made me smile:
....
....
Something I am proud of: ....
....
Something I am grateful for: ....
....
....
Something I am looking forward to: ....
....
....

Lowest pain level today: 1 2 3 4 5
Highest pain level today: 1 2 3 4 5

Wednesday.........................

Sleep rating: 1 2 3 4 5

Mindset goal: ....
....

Eating goal: ....
....

Personal hygiene: bathe ...... teeth ......
style hair ...... get dressed ...... other ......

Pain Management Strategies:

- [ ] deep breathing [ ] meditation
- [ ] visualization [ ] one object focus
- [ ] calming scents [ ] PMR
- [ ] rest [ ] music

Something that made me smile:
....
....
Something I am proud of: ....
....
Something I am grateful for: ....
....
....
Something I am looking forward to: ....
....
....

Lowest pain level today: 1 2 3 4 5
Highest pain level today: 1 2 3 4 5

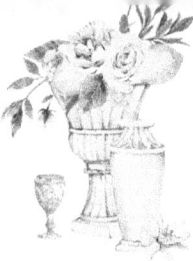

Sleep rating: 1 2 3 4 5

Mindset goal: ....
....

Eating goal: ....
....

Personal hygiene: bathe ...... teeth ......
style hair ...... get dressed ...... other ......

Pain Management Strategies:

- [ ] deep breathing   [ ] meditation
- [ ] visualization   [ ] one object focus
- [ ] calming scents   [ ] PMR
- [ ] rest   [ ] music

Something that made me smile:
....
....

Something I am proud of: ....
....

Something I am grateful for: ....
....

Something I am looking forward to: ....
....

Lowest pain level today: 1 2 3 4 5
Highest pain level today: 1 2 3 4 5

Friday...........................

Sleep rating: 1 2 3 4 5

Mindset goal: ....
....

Eating goal: ....
....

Personal hygiene: bathe ...... teeth ......
style hair ...... get dressed ...... other ......

Pain Management Strategies:

- [ ] deep breathing   [ ] meditation
- [ ] visualization   [ ] one object focus
- [ ] calming scents   [ ] PMR
- [ ] rest   [ ] music

Something that made me smile:
....
....

Something I am proud of: ....
....

Something I am grateful for: ....
....

Something I am looking forward to: ....
....

Lowest pain level today: 1 2 3 4 5
Highest pain level today: 1 2 3 4 5

Saturday

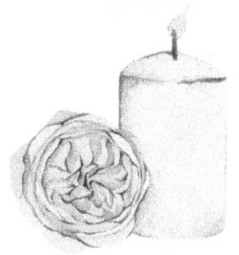

Sleep rating: 1 2 3 4 5

Mindset goal: ....
....

Eating goal: ....
....

Personal hygiene: bathe ......   teeth ......
style hair ......   get dressed ......   other ......

Pain Management Strategies:

- [ ] deep breathing
- [ ] visualization
- [ ] calming scents
- [ ] rest
- [ ] meditation
- [ ] one object focus
- [ ] PMR
- [ ] music

Something that made me smile:
....
....

Something I am proud of: ....
....

Something I am grateful for: ....
....

Something I am looking forward to: ....
....

Lowest pain level today: 1 2 3 4 5
Highest pain level today: 1 2 3 4 5

Sunday

Sleep rating: 1 2 3 4 5

Mindset goal: ....
....

Eating goal: ....
....

Personal hygiene: bathe ......   teeth ......
style hair ......   get dressed ......   other ......

Pain Management Strategies:

- [ ] deep breathing
- [ ] visualization
- [ ] calming scents
- [ ] rest
- [ ] meditation
- [ ] one object focus
- [ ] PMR
- [ ] music

Something that made me smile:
....
....

Something I am proud of: ....
....

Something I am grateful for: ....
....

Something I am looking forward to: ....
....

Lowest pain level today: 1 2 3 4 5
Highest pain level today: 1 2 3 4 5

Monthly Reflection

Think about how your mental health was this month. Did you use the strategies?
When were you your best? Your worst?

....

....

....

....

....

....

....

....

....

....

....

....

....

....

....

....

....

....

Happy Distraction

Draw the other half of this butterfly. No pressure! Just have fun.

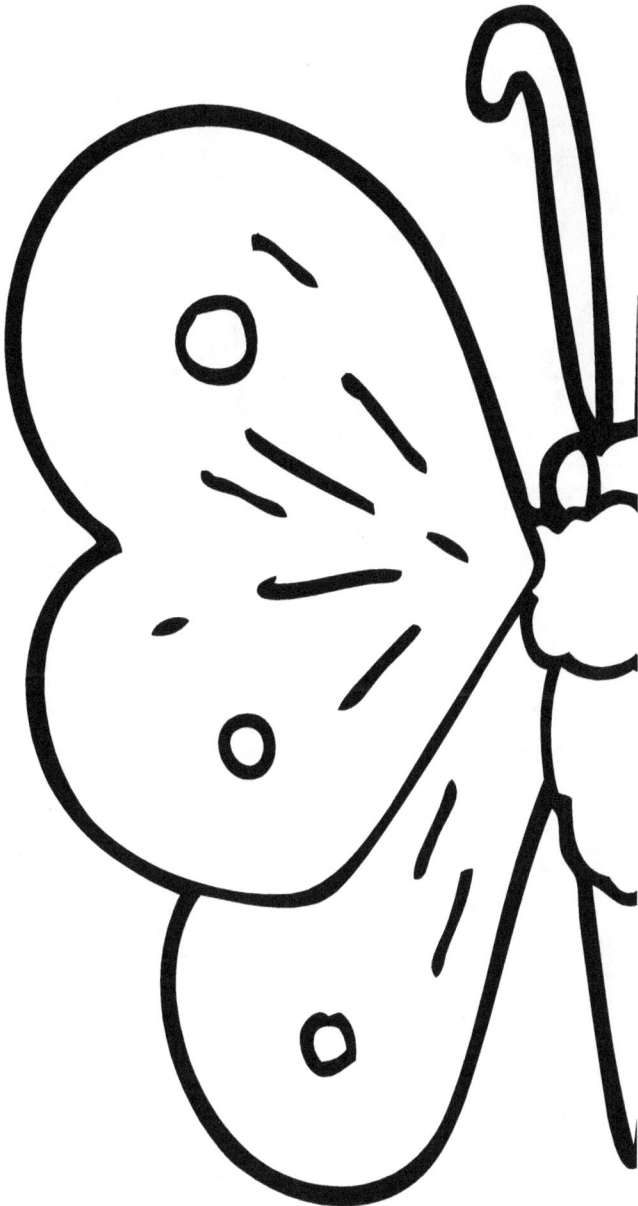

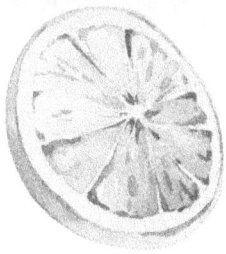

Week Forty-Nine

Goal for the week: ....
....

Days/Times I will leave the house or change settings: ....
....

When I will interact with friends or family: ....
....

Hobby I will work on: ....

Something new I'll try: ....

Medical tasks to do : ....
....
....

Monday.........................

Sleep rating: 1 2 3 4 5

Mindset goal: ....
....

Eating goal: ....
....

Personal hygiene: bathe ...... teeth ......
style hair ...... get dressed ...... other ......

Pain Management Strategies:

☐ deep breathing ☐ meditation
☐ visualization ☐ one object focus
☐ calming scents ☐ PMR
☐ rest ☐ music

Something that made me smile:
....
....
Something I am proud of: ....
....
Something I am grateful for: ....
....
Something I am looking forward to: ....
....
....

Lowest pain level today: 1 2 3 4 5
Highest pain level today: 1 2 3 4 5

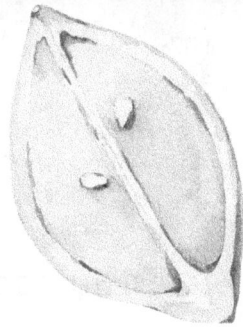

Week Forty-Nine

Tuesday......................

Sleep rating: 1 2 3 4 5

Mindset goal: ....
....

Eating goal: ....
....

Personal hygiene: bathe ......   teeth ......
style hair ......   get dressed ......   other ......

Pain Management Strategies:

☐ deep breathing ☐ meditation
☐ visualization   ☐ one object focus
☐ calming scents ☐ PMR
☐ rest   ☐ music

Something that made me smile:
....
....
Something I am proud of: ....
....
Something I am grateful for: ....
....
Something I am looking forward to: ....
....

Lowest pain level today: 1 2 3 4 5
Highest pain level today: 1 2 3 4 5

Wednesday.........................

Sleep rating: 1 2 3 4 5

Mindset goal: ....
....

Eating goal: ....
....

Personal hygiene: bathe ......   teeth ......
style hair ......   get dressed ......   other ......

Pain Management Strategies:

☐ deep breathing ☐ meditation
☐ visualization   ☐ one object focus
☐ calming scents ☐ PMR
☐ rest   ☐ music

Something that made me smile:
....
....
Something I am proud of: ....
....
Something I am grateful for: ....
....
Something I am looking forward to: ....
....

Lowest pain level today: 1 2 3 4 5
Highest pain level today: 1 2 3 4 5

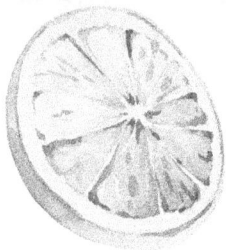

Week Forty-Nine

Thursday..................

Sleep rating: 1 2 3 4 5

Mindset goal: ....
....

Eating goal: ....
....

Personal hygiene: bathe ...... teeth ......
style hair ...... get dressed ...... other ......

Pain Management Strategies:

☐ deep breathing ☐ meditation
☐ visualization ☐ one object focus
☐ calming scents ☐ PMR
☐ rest ☐ music

Something that made me smile:
....
....
Something I am proud of: ....
....
Something I am grateful for: ....
....
Something I am looking forward to: ....
....
....
Lowest pain level today: 1 2 3 4 5
Highest pain level today: 1 2 3 4 5

Friday.........................

Sleep rating: 1 2 3 4 5

Mindset goal: ....
....

Eating goal: ....
....

Personal hygiene: bathe ...... teeth ......
style hair ...... get dressed ...... other ......

Pain Management Strategies:

☐ deep breathing ☐ meditation
☐ visualization ☐ one object focus
☐ calming scents ☐ PMR
☐ rest ☐ music

Something that made me smile:
....
....
Something I am proud of: ....
....
Something I am grateful for: ....
....
Something I am looking forward to: ....
....
....
Lowest pain level today: 1 2 3 4 5
Highest pain level today: 1 2 3 4 5

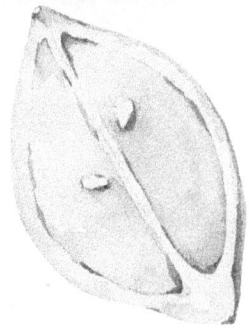

Week Forty-Nine

Saturday.....................

Sleep rating: 1 2 3 4 5

Mindset goal: ....
....

Eating goal: ....
....

Personal hygiene: bathe ...... teeth ......
style hair ...... get dressed ...... other ......

Pain Management Strategies:

- [ ] deep breathing
- [ ] visualization
- [ ] calming scents
- [ ] rest
- [ ] meditation
- [ ] one object focus
- [ ] PMR
- [ ] music

Something that made me smile:
....
....
Something I am proud of: ....
....
Something I am grateful for: ....
....
Something I am looking forward to: ....
....
Lowest pain level today: 1 2 3 4 5
Highest pain level today: 1 2 3 4 5

Sunday........................

Sleep rating: 1 2 3 4 5

Mindset goal: ....
....

Eating goal: ....
....

Personal hygiene: bathe ...... teeth ......
style hair ...... get dressed ...... other ......

Pain Management Strategies:

- [ ] deep breathing
- [ ] visualization
- [ ] calming scents
- [ ] rest
- [ ] meditation
- [ ] one object focus
- [ ] PMR
- [ ] music

Something that made me smile:
....
....
Something I am proud of: ....
....
Something I am grateful for: ....
....
Something I am looking forward to: ....
....
Lowest pain level today: 1 2 3 4 5
Highest pain level today: 1 2 3 4 5

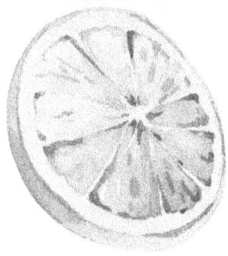

Week Fifty

Goal for the week: ....
....

Days/Times I will leave the house or change settings: ....
....

When I will interact with friends or family: ....
....

Hobby I will work on: ....

Something new I'll try: ....

Medical tasks to do : ....
....
....

Monday.........................

Sleep rating: 1 2 3 4 5

Mindset goal: ....
....

Eating goal: ....
....

Personal hygiene: bathe ......   teeth ......
style hair ......   get dressed ......   other ......

Pain Management Strategies:

☐ deep breathing ☐ meditation
☐ visualization   ☐ one object focus
☐ calming scents ☐ PMR
☐ rest   ☐ music

Something that made me smile:
....
....

Something I am proud of: ....
....

Something I am grateful for: ....
....

Something I am looking forward to: ....
....
....

Lowest pain level today: 1 2 3 4 5
Highest pain level today: 1 2 3 4 5

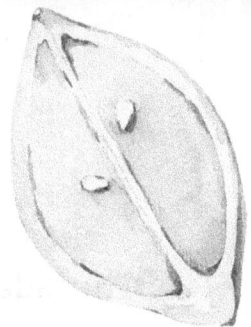

Week Fifty

Tuesday........................

Sleep rating: 1 2 3 4 5

Mindset goal: ....
....

Eating goal: ....
....

Personal hygiene: bathe ...... teeth ......
style hair ...... get dressed ...... other ......

Pain Management Strategies:

☐ deep breathing ☐ meditation
☐ visualization ☐ one object focus
☐ calming scents ☐ PMR
☐ rest ☐ music

Something that made me smile:
....
....

Something I am proud of: ....
....

Something I am grateful for: ....
....

Something I am looking forward to: ....
....

Lowest pain level today: 1 2 3 4 5
Highest pain level today: 1 2 3 4 5

Wednesday..........................

Sleep rating: 1 2 3 4 5

Mindset goal: ....
....

Eating goal: ....
....

Personal hygiene: bathe ...... teeth ......
style hair ...... get dressed ...... other ......

Pain Management Strategies:

☐ deep breathing ☐ meditation
☐ visualization ☐ one object focus
☐ calming scents ☐ PMR
☐ rest ☐ music

Something that made me smile:
....
....

Something I am proud of: ....
....

Something I am grateful for: ....
....

Something I am looking forward to: ....
....

Lowest pain level today: 1 2 3 4 5
Highest pain level today: 1 2 3 4 5

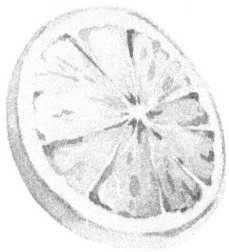

Thursday..................... Week Fifty

Sleep rating: 1 2 3 4 5

Mindset goal: ....
....

Eating goal: ....
....

Personal hygiene: bathe ......   teeth ......
style hair ......   get dressed ......   other ......

Pain Management Strategies:

- [ ] deep breathing
- [ ] visualization
- [ ] calming scents
- [ ] rest
- [ ] meditation
- [ ] one object focus
- [ ] PMR
- [ ] music

Something that made me smile:
....
....

Something I am proud of: ....

Something I am grateful for: ....

Something I am looking forward to: ....
....
....

Lowest pain level today: 1 2 3 4 5
Highest pain level today: 1 2 3 4 5

Friday.........................

Sleep rating: 1 2 3 4 5

Mindset goal: ....
....

Eating goal: ....
....

Personal hygiene: bathe ......   teeth ......
style hair ......   get dressed ......   other ......

Pain Management Strategies:

- [ ] deep breathing
- [ ] visualization
- [ ] calming scents
- [ ] rest
- [ ] meditation
- [ ] one object focus
- [ ] PMR
- [ ] music

Something that made me smile:
....
....

Something I am proud of: ....

Something I am grateful for: ....

Something I am looking forward to: ....
....
....

Lowest pain level today: 1 2 3 4 5
Highest pain level today: 1 2 3 4 5

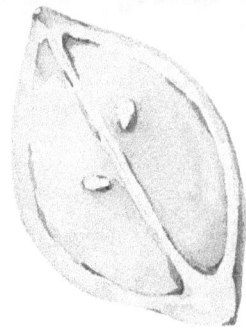

Saturday..................... Week Fifty

Sleep rating: 1 2 3 4 5

Mindset goal: ....
....

Eating goal: ....
....

Personal hygiene: bathe ......   teeth ......
style hair ......   get dressed ......   other ......

Pain Management Strategies:

☐ deep breathing   ☐ meditation
☐ visualization   ☐ one object focus
☐ calming scents   ☐ PMR
☐ rest   ☐ music

Something that made me smile:
....
....

Something I am proud of: ....

Something I am grateful for: ....

Something I am looking forward to: ....
....
....

Lowest pain level today: 1 2 3 4 5
Highest pain level today: 1 2 3 4 5

Sunday.........................

Sleep rating: 1 2 3 4 5

Mindset goal: ....
....

Eating goal: ....
....

Personal hygiene: bathe ......   teeth ......
style hair ......   get dressed ......   other ......

Pain Management Strategies:

☐ deep breathing   ☐ meditation
☐ visualization   ☐ one object focus
☐ calming scents   ☐ PMR
☐ rest   ☐ music

Something that made me smile:
....
....

Something I am proud of: ....

Something I am grateful for: ....

Something I am looking forward to: ....
....
....

Lowest pain level today: 1 2 3 4 5
Highest pain level today: 1 2 3 4 5

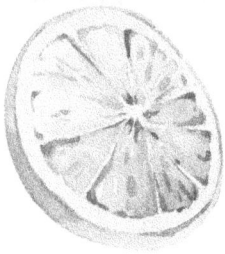

Week Fifty-One

Goal for the week: ....
....

Days/Times I will leave the house or change settings: ....
....

When I will interact with friends or family: ....
....

Hobby I will work on: ....

Something new I'll try: ....

Medical tasks to do : ....
....
....

Monday.........................

Sleep rating: 1 2 3 4 5

Mindset goal: ....
....

Eating goal: ....
....

Personal hygiene: bathe ...... teeth ......
style hair ...... get dressed ...... other ......

Pain Management Strategies:

- [ ] deep breathing
- [ ] visualization
- [ ] calming scents
- [ ] rest
- [ ] meditation
- [ ] one object focus
- [ ] PMR
- [ ] music

Something that made me smile:
....
....

Something I am proud of: ....
....

Something I am grateful for: ....
....

Something I am looking forward to: ....
....
....

Lowest pain level today: 1 2 3 4 5
Highest pain level today: 1 2 3 4 5

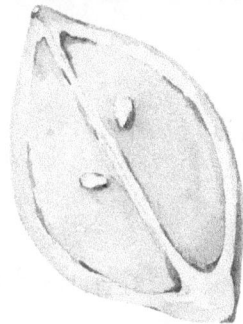

Tuesday..........................

Sleep rating: 1 2 3 4 5

Mindset goal: ....

....

Eating goal: ....

....

Personal hygiene: bathe ...... teeth ......
style hair ...... get dressed ...... other ......

Pain Management Strategies:

- [ ] deep breathing
- [ ] visualization
- [ ] calming scents
- [ ] rest
- [ ] meditation
- [ ] one object focus
- [ ] PMR
- [ ] music

Something that made me smile:

....

....

Something I am proud of: ....

....

Something I am grateful for: ....

....

Something I am looking forward to: ....

....

Lowest pain level today: 1 2 3 4 5
Highest pain level today: 1 2 3 4 5

Wednesday...........................

Sleep rating: 1 2 3 4 5

Mindset goal: ....

....

Eating goal: ....

....

Personal hygiene: bathe ...... teeth ......
style hair ...... get dressed ...... other ......

Pain Management Strategies:

- [ ] deep breathing
- [ ] visualization
- [ ] calming scents
- [ ] rest
- [ ] meditation
- [ ] one object focus
- [ ] PMR
- [ ] music

Something that made me smile:

....

....

Something I am proud of: ....

....

Something I am grateful for: ....

....

....

Something I am looking forward to: ....

....

....

Lowest pain level today: 1 2 3 4 5
Highest pain level today: 1 2 3 4 5

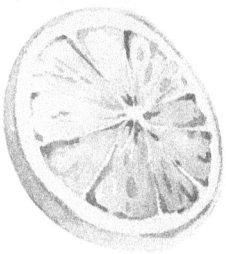

Thursday.................... *Week Fifty-One*

Sleep rating: 1 2 3 4 5

Mindset goal: ....
....

Eating goal: ....
....

Personal hygiene: bathe ...... teeth ......
style hair ...... get dressed ...... other ......

Pain Management Strategies:

☐ deep breathing ☐ meditation
☐ visualization ☐ one object focus
☐ calming scents ☐ PMR
☐ rest ☐ music

Something that made me smile:
....
....

Something I am proud of: ....
....

Something I am grateful for: ....
....

Something I am looking forward to: ....
....
....

Lowest pain level today: 1 2 3 4 5
Highest pain level today: 1 2 3 4 5

Friday.........................

Sleep rating: 1 2 3 4 5

Mindset goal: ....
....

Eating goal: ....
....

Personal hygiene: bathe ...... teeth ......
style hair ...... get dressed ...... other ......

Pain Management Strategies:

☐ deep breathing ☐ meditation
☐ visualization ☐ one object focus
☐ calming scents ☐ PMR
☐ rest ☐ music

Something that made me smile:
....
....

Something I am proud of: ....
....

Something I am grateful for: ....
....

Something I am looking forward to: ....
....
....

Lowest pain level today: 1 2 3 4 5
Highest pain level today: 1 2 3 4 5

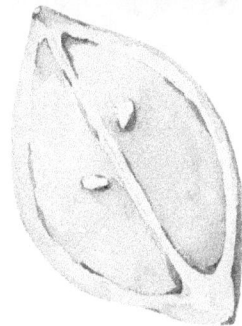

Week Fifty-One

Saturday.....................

Sleep rating: 1 2 3 4 5

Mindset goal: ....
....

Eating goal: ....
....

Personal hygiene: bathe ......   teeth ......
style hair ......   get dressed ......   other ......

Pain Management Strategies:

☐ deep breathing ☐ meditation
☐ visualization ☐ one object focus
☐ calming scents ☐ PMR
☐ rest ☐ music

Something that made me smile:
....
....

Something I am proud of: ....
....

Something I am grateful for: ....
....

Something I am looking forward to: ....
....

Lowest pain level today: 1 2 3 4 5
Highest pain level today: 1 2 3 4 5

Sunday........................

Sleep rating: 1 2 3 4 5

Mindset goal: ....
....

Eating goal: ....
....

Personal hygiene: bathe ......   teeth ......
style hair ......   get dressed ......   other ......

Pain Management Strategies:

☐ deep breathing ☐ meditation
☐ visualization ☐ one object focus
☐ calming scents ☐ PMR
☐ rest ☐ music

Something that made me smile:
....
....

Something I am proud of: ....
....

Something I am grateful for: ....
....

Something I am looking forward to: ....
....

Lowest pain level today: 1 2 3 4 5
Highest pain level today: 1 2 3 4 5

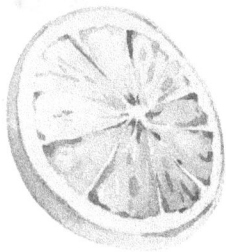

Week Fifty-Two

Goal for the week: ....
....

Days/Times I will leave the house or change settings: ....
....

When I will interact with friends or family: ....
....

Hobby I will work on: ....

Something new I'll try: ....

Medical tasks to do : ....
....
....

Monday..........................

Sleep rating: 1   2   3   4   5

Mindset goal: ....
....

Eating goal: ....
....

Personal hygiene: bathe ......   teeth ......
style hair ......   get dressed ......   other ......

Pain Management Strategies:

- [ ] deep breathing [ ] meditation
- [ ] visualization [ ] one object focus
- [ ] calming scents [ ] PMR
- [ ] rest [ ] music

Something that made me smile:
....
....
Something I am proud of: ....
....
Something I am grateful for: ....
....
Something I am looking forward to: ....
....
....

Lowest pain level today: 1 2 3 4 5
Highest pain level today: 1 2 3 4 5

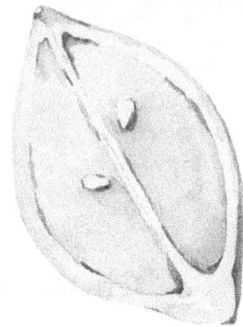

Tuesday........................ *Week Fifty-Two*

Sleep rating: 1 2 3 4 5

Mindset goal: ....
....

Eating goal: ....
....

Personal hygiene: bathe ......   teeth ......
style hair ......   get dressed ......   other ......

Pain Management Strategies:

☐ deep breathing   ☐ meditation
☐ visualization   ☐ one object focus
☐ calming scents   ☐ PMR
☐ rest   ☐ music

Something that made me smile:
....
....

Something I am proud of: ....
....

Something I am grateful for: ....
....

Something I am looking forward to: ....
....
....

Lowest pain level today: 1 2 3 4 5
Highest pain level today: 1 2 3 4 5

Wednesday........................

Sleep rating: 1 2 3 4 5

Mindset goal: ....
....

Eating goal: ....
....

Personal hygiene: bathe ......   teeth ......
style hair ......   get dressed ......   other ......

Pain Management Strategies:

☐ deep breathing   ☐ meditation
☐ visualization   ☐ one object focus
☐ calming scents   ☐ PMR
☐ rest   ☐ music

Something that made me smile:
....
....

Something I am proud of: ....
....

Something I am grateful for: ....
....

Something I am looking forward to: ....
....
....

Lowest pain level today: 1 2 3 4 5
Highest pain level today: 1 2 3 4 5

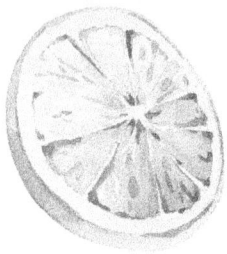

Thursday......................... *Week Fifty-Two*

Sleep rating: 1 2 3 4 5

Mindset goal: ....
....

Eating goal: ....
....

Personal hygiene: bathe ...... teeth ......
style hair ...... get dressed ...... other ......

Pain Management Strategies:

☐ deep breathing ☐ meditation
☐ visualization ☐ one object focus
☐ calming scents ☐ PMR
☐ rest ☐ music

Something that made me smile:
....
....

Something I am proud of: ....
....

Something I am grateful for: ....
....

Something I am looking forward to: ....
....
....

Lowest pain level today: 1 2 3 4 5
Highest pain level today: 1 2 3 4 5

Friday.........................

Sleep rating: 1 2 3 4 5

Mindset goal: ....
....

Eating goal: ....
....

Personal hygiene: bathe ...... teeth ......
style hair ...... get dressed ...... other ......

Pain Management Strategies:

☐ deep breathing ☐ meditation
☐ visualization ☐ one object focus
☐ calming scents ☐ PMR
☐ rest ☐ music

Something that made me smile:
....
....

Something I am proud of: ....
....

Something I am grateful for: ....
....

Something I am looking forward to: ....
....
....

Lowest pain level today: 1 2 3 4 5
Highest pain level today: 1 2 3 4 5

Saturday...................... *Week Fifty-Two*

Sleep rating: 1 2 3 4 5

Mindset goal: ....
....

Eating goal: ....
....

Personal hygiene: bathe ...... teeth ......
style hair ...... get dressed ...... other ......

Pain Management Strategies:

- [ ] deep breathing [ ] meditation
- [ ] visualization [ ] one object focus
- [ ] calming scents [ ] PMR
- [ ] rest [ ] music

Something that made me smile:
....
....
Something I am proud of: ....
....
Something I am grateful for: ....
....
Something I am looking forward to: ....
....
....
Lowest pain level today: 1 2 3 4 5
Highest pain level today: 1 2 3 4 5

Sunday.........................

Sleep rating: 1 2 3 4 5

Mindset goal: ....
....

Eating goal: ....
....

Personal hygiene: bathe ...... teeth ......
style hair ...... get dressed ...... other ......

Pain Management Strategies:

- [ ] deep breathing [ ] meditation
- [ ] visualization [ ] one object focus
- [ ] calming scents [ ] PMR
- [ ] rest [ ] music

Something that made me smile:
....
....
Something I am proud of: ....
....
Something I am grateful for: ....
....
....
Something I am looking forward to: ....
....
....
Lowest pain level today: 1 2 3 4 5
Highest pain level today: 1 2 3 4 5

Closing Reflections

Take a moment to reflect on your year and your health journey. What were your high points? Low points? What strategies helped you the most?

....

....

....

....

....

....

....

....

....

....

....

Closing Reflections

....

....

....

....

....

....

....

....

....

....

....

....

Goals For Next Year

....
....
....
....
....
....
....
....
....
....
....
....
....
....
....
....
....
....

Goals For Next Year

....
....
....
....
....
....
....
....
....
....
....
....
....
....
....
....
....

Other Journals from Orange Blossom

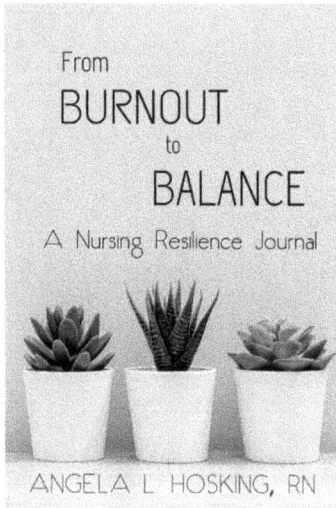

From Burnout to Balance:
A Nursing Resilience Journal

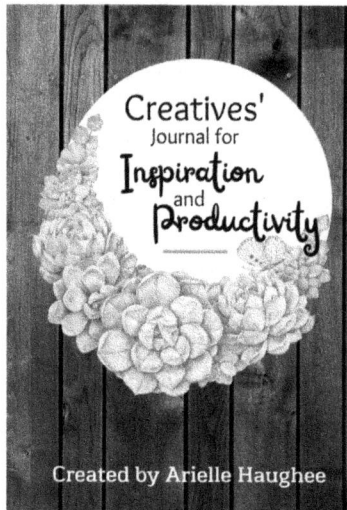

Creatives' Journal for
Inspiration and Productivity

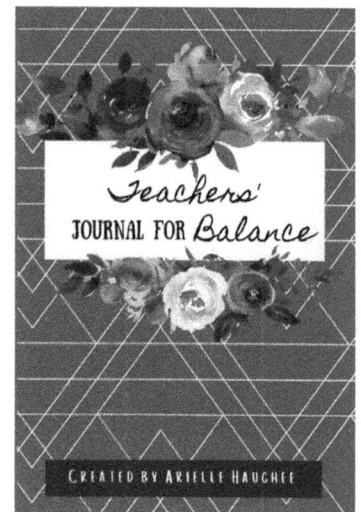

Teachers' Journal for
Balance

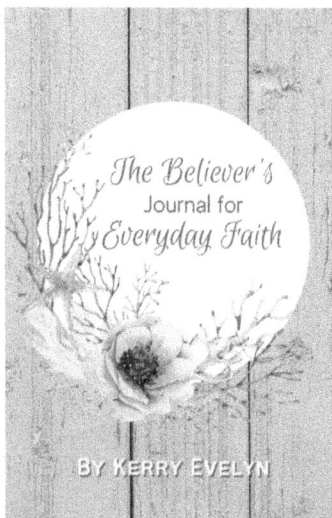

The Believer's Journal for
Everyday Faith

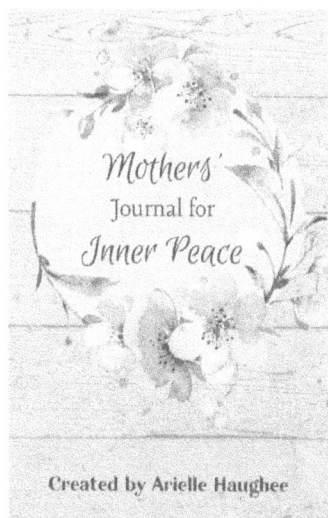

Mothers' Journal for
Inner Peace

Scan here to see the
journals and other
great books!

www.ingramcontent.com/pod-product-compliance
Lightning Source LLC
Chambersburg PA
CBHW080417030426
42335CB00020B/2483